Quincy

Janet P. Bailey

Copyright © 2013 by Janet P. Bailey

This book is a work of fiction. Names, characters, places, and incidents are the product of the author's imagination or are used fictitiously.

All Rights Reserved. In accordance with the U.S. Copyright Act of 1976, the scanning, uploading, and electronic sharing of any part of this book without the permission of the author constitute unlawful piracy and theft of the author's intellectual property.

Thank you for your support of the author's rights.

Except for the original material written by the author, all speeches are property of the respective writers and copyright holders.

ISBN:978-1494342869

Chapter 1

Sara walked down the long, concrete ramp, through the heavy metal doors and into the large animal clinic at the University of Tennessee, College of Veterinary Medicine. A March breeze was blowing through the entrance corridor, and the scent of disinfectant mixed with manure wafted through the air.

A young calf was balling for its mother at the far end of the food animal ward while the clip clop of horses' hooves could be heard resounding off the cinder block walls as patients in the equine ward were being led outside for morning turnout.

Sara closed her eyes and inhaled deeply. These were the smells and sounds of rural Tennessee where she had been born and raised. These were memories of home, and after last night, she needed these reminders to calm her nerves and still her racing brain.

As a fourth year veterinary student in the large animal internal medicine rotation, it had been Sara's turn for emergency call last night. March is a very busy time in veterinary practice. Just about every farm species is having babies or trying to, and along with babies, come problems - big problems. Veterinarians know a different side of the miracle of birth, and it's not what one sees in the movies or reads in books.

Sometimes, the cow doesn't always easily have the calf in a well-bedded stall, and, even then, she doesn't always turn to nuzzle and love on her newborn. The mare doesn't always believe that her foal is the most wonderful thing on earth, and the foal doesn't always stand shortly after birth on its wobbly legs to look at its mother with those big, brown eyes.

Things can, at times, go very wrong, and that's what veterinarians see. That is also what Sara saw last night, and every time she had tried to get some sleep, the emergency cell phone attached to her belt would vibrate. More work needed to be done. More mares needed help and more foals needed attention. More cows were having trouble, and more calves needed her fledgling expertise.

By the time the morning light had finally begun seeping its way into the small windows and under the large roll up doors of the facility at six a.m., Sara was exhausted. She had been able to catch an hour nap on the old cot in the break room before getting up at seven to treat her patients and prepare for morning rounds.

Rounds at eight had gone off without a hitch, and before her first appointment at nine, Sara had even had time to slide on another pair of university issued puke green coveralls, re-tie her black unruly hair back into a ponytail, and wash the smudged mascara from under her brown eyes. It was ten till nine and her turn again. The next client was waiting. Sara sighed, walked into the exam room and forced a smile for Mrs. Taylor.

Judy Taylor had left home with her horse, Quincy, at one am this morning. The haul from Memphis to Knoxville usually ran six to seven hours, and with the time change and their appointment being at nine, she wanted to make sure they were on time. She, too, was exhausted.

Quincy had been sick on and off for two years, but in the last two weeks, he had gotten much worse. She had done everything her veterinarian had prescribed, but nothing seemed to make Quincy better. Her vet had told her it was time for Quincy to either go to a specialist or for Judy to consider euthanasia. Judy knew Quincy might never come home if she brought him to Knoxville, but the thought of putting him down had been too much for her to bear. So, here she finally was waiting in the exam room for the specialist, but instead, a young girl walks into the room.

"Hi, Mrs. Taylor, my name is Sara Caldwell, and I'll be the student on Quincy's case. You mind if I ask you a couple of questions about him before we start the exam?" Sara asked as she extended her hand to Judy.

"Not at all, Hon, but when's the doctor coming in?" Judy asked as she took Sara's young hand sizing her up in the process. Sara's handshake was firm, like handshakes should be - even from a woman.

Judy knew Sara had been around horses all her life. Horse people knew other horse people when they saw them. It was just one of those things. Judy liked Sara already.

"Dr. Sneed will be in after me and Dr. Summers take a look at him, Mrs. Taylor. I just need to get a couple of things straight about the history of his illness, and then we'll go from there." Sara replied.

As Sara thumbed through Quincy's medical record asking Judy questions, Sara was doing a little sizing up of her own. Sara had seen clients bring horses who were only worried about the next race, the next event, the next big check, and no matter how sick or crippled the horse might be, they wanted it to run or work again so they could collect their money. Judy didn't seem like this type of horse owner, but Sara had been fooled before.

Judy also had a superior air about her that comes from having lots of money, something Sara knew nothing about. Most of their clients here at the referral hospital didn't have to worry about money. Veterinary care wasn't cheap and when you threw in specialty care, round the clock service, and the best diagnostic tools available, the care here was anything but inexpensive.

From Judy's designer boots and clothes to the diamonds she wore on her ears and fingers, Sara knew this woman had lots of money. Sara also knew that people with this type of wealth were used to getting what they wanted when they wanted it and that could cause problems in client relations. Sometimes it just didn't matter how much money you had, some patients couldn't be fixed.

When Sara had finished sizing Judy up, asked all the questions she had been taught to ask, and recorded the answers in Quincy's record, she closed the medical record, and asked Judy to bring him in. It was time to do the physical exam.

Chapter 2

Judy thought the student was never going to stop asking questions. She knew it was Sara's job, but she also knew Quincy had not done well with the trailer ride. When she had arrived in Knoxville, she'd peeked into the trailer. He didn't look well. She was just glad to finally unload him.

Judy untied the lead rope from the front of the trailer, opened the back doors, and brought down the safety bar to clue Quincy they were finally there, and he could back out. As Quincy unloaded, he stumbled a little, and for a moment, Judy was afraid he might fall. He was just working so hard to breathe. Quincy steadied himself, and Judy slowly led him into the room for Sara to examine.

Sara heard Quincy before he ever entered the room. From the sound of his hooves slowly dragging across the pavement in the unloading area to the loud unnatural wheeze every time he took a breath, Sara knew this horse was sick before she ever laid eyes on him.

When Sara saw him for the first time, all exhaustion vanished. The cobwebs that had been gathering in Sara's brain because of sleep and food deprivation were cleared. It was time to go to work. This guy needed some serious help.

Quincy had once been a big horse, that was obvious from his frame, but he had been sick for a while. Disease had stolen most of his muscle and fat, and at first look, Sara thought maybe his spirit. He was a Thoroughbred, but unlike many of his breed, Sara could tell by his intelligent eyes that Quincy was a gentle giant even when he had been healthy and strong.

He stood 17 hands tall, a once beautiful horse with a burnished red head and body. His jet-black mane and tail stood in contrast to the white markings on all four legs and the big blaze that reached from his eyes down to his nose. Sara imagined that before he had gotten sick, people stopped in their tracks to stare at him. He would have been that beautiful. If people saw him now, they would stare for a different reason.

Sara also noticed Judy as she led her horse into the room. Judy was gently urging Quincy to take one more step, one more. While Judy was leading Quincy with one hand, the other was placed on the side of his neck to let him know she was right there, and she would help him if needed. Sara also noticed the tears streaming down Judy's face and her previous doubts about this woman were forgotten. Judy was here for her horse, and as Sara watched Judy will Quincy to take another step, one thing was clear - Judy loved Quincy and would give anything to have him well again.

"That's good right there, Mrs. Taylor. That's far enough. We'll let him rest a minute while I look at him," Sara said as she took the lead rope from Judy and begin rubbing the big blaze on Quincy's face.

"This boy's had it rough already today. There's no reason to bring him further in the room. We'll let him catch his breath."

"Okay, Sara, I think he would appreciate that. I know you must think I'm either insane or just plain cruel to bring him all this way in his condition, but he won't give up. I can see it in his eyes, and until he gives up, I've got to try everything I can to make him better. I just can't let him down. I love him dearly, Sara, and I sure hope y'all can help him."

"Well, Mrs. Taylor, we'll sure try - I promise you that." Sara looked into Mrs. Taylor's eyes and the pain and worry she saw there made her feel for this woman, but she couldn't show any emotion. She was supposed to be the professional, and therefore, she had to maintain a professional demeanor.

Sara took a deep breath to gain composure and then, almost with machine like precision, she began to examine Quincy.

Chapter 3

Sara had always been able to process information from many different sources at one time. If she had to describe this little talent of hers, she would say she had many voices inside her head talking about different things but all making sense, and not in the schizophrenic way. Sara found it slightly peculiar that since she had been in vet school, there was a time when all the voices inside her head would become silent - except one.

It was a very calm voice that was unbiased, unemotional, and processed information with expediency and confidence. That voice only spoke to Sara when she was examining an animal. All other sights, sounds, and sensory stimuli seemed to fade far into the background. Only the voice and what it saw, felt or heard through the stethoscope mattered. Sara had come to trust and listen to that voice.

On Quincy's exam, the calm voice inside her head was not very hopeful. From Quincy's history, Sara already knew this horse had been diagnosed with COPD and had been receiving treatment for years. Sara also knew, from her many hours in the classroom that COPD in horses was much the same as in people. The disease attacked the lungs and airways making it difficult, at times, to even take a single breath.

As she did her exam, the voice told Sara that Quincy's particular condition was very advanced, that the lungs were severely compromised and the rest of the body was suffering. Sara's voice told her, in no uncertain terms, that this guy was in bad shape and extreme measures were needed. Her voice also told her that Quincy's chances of improving were slim to none no matter what they did.

Sara finished with her exam, and as the voice became quiet, Sara looked into Quincy's eyes. In those eyes, she saw a tremendous amount of pain but also a tremendous will to live, and she saw hope.

In those eyes, Sara saw a plea for help, a plea to be able to breathe deeply again, to be able to run again, to be able to spend more time with Judy, his friend.

For the first time in her young career, Sara found that it really didn't matter what that calm voice inside her head had said, she needed to make this horse better, and she needed to reassure him that she could. Miracles did happen. Sara had seen several here in this hospital. Quincy would be one of hers.

Sara smiled, and as she reached for Quincy to stroke and reassure him, he placed his head on Sara's shoulder. He let out a shuddering sigh. Judy began to laugh.

"He likes you Sara. That's what he does now when he likes somebody. When he was healthy, I would go to the barn every morning to ride. I would open his stall door, and he would come up to me, put that head down by my knee and run it all the way up to my shoulder where he would just rest for a minute. He was so strong. I always had to brace myself so he wouldn't knock me down. Since he's been sick, though, I think he only has the energy to just rest it on my shoulder. He only does that now when he's happy or he knows you understand what he wants. That's a good sign, Sara. Looks like he trusts you. You two will get along fine."

"I think we'll get along fine, too, Mrs. Taylor. He's really quite a guy, isn't he?" Sara asked. "Now, if you'll stay with him, I'm going to step out a minute and get the resident, and I'll be right back. Just try to keep him as comfortable as possible while I'm gone."

Sara handed Quincy's lead rope back to Mrs. Taylor, gave her a sympathetic touch on the shoulder, and left the room.

Back up the hall, through the doors, and into the break room Sara went with Quincy's file in hand. The rapid fire questioning would begin as soon as Sara stepped into the room, and she needed a minute to compose herself. Her emotions seemed to be on overdrive with this horse.

The little cobwebs were returning as she tried to remember everything she knew about COPD. She needed to be ready for the upcoming inquisition by the resident on rotation, Dr. Julia Summers.

If clinical rotations taught you anything, they taught you to think quickly under pressure and function even when you were exhausted.

Sara took a minute outside the break room to gather all her thoughts. She readied herself and entered the room. Dr. Summers was drinking her second cup of espresso, looking over the charts from morning rounds, and waiting for Sara's presentation of the case.

Chapter 4

Dr. Julia Summers was now in her second year of a three-year residency. Her life ambition was to be an equine specialist and not just a mediocre one- she wanted to be one of the best. She was 5'3 with long blonde hair, and soaking wet, she might weigh 100 pounds - all of which was muscle and grit. She was a petite woman with anything but a petite attitude when it came to doing her job, teaching these students a thing or two about horses, and following her dreams.

She was compassionate and reasonable, and demanded no more from her students than she would expect from herself which most of the time, was a hundred and ten percent. In the three weeks Sara had been on this rotation, she had come to admire and trust Dr. Summers. Sara just hoped she could be half the veterinarian Dr. Summers was one day.

Julia had also come to admire Sara in the detached way most residents view students. She had taught Sara throughout the four-week rotation, and they were on their last week. Julia had found Sara to be a worker with a desire to learn and a deep compassion for the animals she treated. Students like Sara made Julia's job much easier.

Still, Julia kept a very close eye on all the students in her rotation. It was imperative for two reasons. First, the students took care of her patients, and she wanted to make sure her patients were treated correctly and with care. Second, the attitudes of the students could make a world of difference in how they worked individually and together as a team.

Because of her close supervision, Julia knew Sara had been up all night with incoming patients. She knew she would be tired, but that was part of the job. If Sara was interested in equine practice when she graduated from here, and she was, she had better learn to perform on limited sleep.

Julia recognized the carefully covered exhaustion on Sara's face when Sara walked into the room. She, too, had seen it many times when looking back at herself from the mirror after long nights on call. There was something new in Sara's face that Julia had not seen before, and it looked a lot like worry.

Julia wondered if Sara was threatened about the questions she would soon ask. As soon as Sara opened her mouth, Julia knew it wasn't her questions, but Sara's patient Sara was worried about.

"Dr. Summers, I've taken a look at Mrs. Taylor's horse, Quincy, and he's pretty sick. He has a two- year history of COPD and has been on every medication available. The trip here was rough on him, and he looks pretty bad. I don't think he's going to make it very long."

"Let's start from the beginning, Sara. Tell me about his history and your physical exam, and we'll go from there."

Sara went through all her findings trying not to leave out any important facts. Julia quizzed Sara on the disease, causative factors, different treatments, and possible outcomes. Sara answered most questions correctly, but by the time Julia had finished her onslaught, Sara had several things she would be looking up before afternoon rounds.

That's the way it always worked. They quizzed you until you got to the point you were just standing there with a blank look on your face saying, "I don't know," over and over. Your grade on the rotation was dependent on your work ethic and how many questions it took one to get to the point of the blank face and the "I don't know" because with every student and every case, the residents and the specialists took you there. That was how you learned.

After Julia felt Sara had been grilled sufficiently, she got up from her chair, slung her stethoscope around her neck, left her much needed espresso on the table, and gestured to Sara that she was ready to take a look at Quincy. The women exited the break room and started down the hall.

"So, this guy does sound like he's in pretty bad shape, Sara."

"Dr. Summers, I know I still have a lot to learn, but I don't think this guy's in pretty bad shape - I know he is. You'll see when we get down there. He's having a hard time breathing."

"How's the client? Is she pretty good or do we have a rough one?"

"I like her. She's the type of person that's used to getting what she wants. It's not going to sit well with her that Dr. Sneed probably won't even look at her horse, but I don't blame her. I'd be demanding, too, if that were my horse." Sara informed Dr. Summers.

"Don't you think just this once he could come down and look at a patient?" Sara asked knowing the answer. "This isn't just a horse to her. He's a good friend."

During the rotation so far, Sara had seen Dr. Sneed only once. It hadn't been a pleasant meeting.

He had shown up one morning for rounds and made her and the other four students in the rotation feel like idiots. It wouldn't have been so bad except Sara could tell he was enjoying putting them all in their place. He wasn't doing it to teach or help them. He just wanted to show his superiority.

Dr. Sneed was a genius, but he was also a very arrogant man who as far as Sara could tell, cared nothing for his patients. He was too deep into research and furthering his career to bother with the mundane dealings of actually becoming interested or treating any of the animals that had come to the hospital under his rotation.

So far, Dr. Sneed had been a voice coming down from above through Dr. Summers, and not only did Sara not care for him, she actually feared him. One bad grade on a rotation, and vet school was over.

"Sara, you know Dr. Sneed is busy with other things and probably won't make it down."

"I know, but this lady has hauled this horse across the state to see him, and I can tell in her eyes that she won't leave until she does. Dr. Sneed is why she's come. I'm pretty sure she's going to insist he look at Quincy."

"Well, we'll deal with that when we have to," answered Dr. Summers.

Chapter 5

Sara and Julia went into the exam room, and Julia introduced herself as Dr. Summers. She asked Judy a couple more questions and also did a physical exam while checking Sara's findings as she went.

All the while, Sara held Quincy and rubbed that spot right under his chin that most horses find pleasant. Quincy rested his head on Sara's shoulder. Judy stood back patiently watching and waiting.

When Julia finished her physical, she turned to Judy and began explaining some of the diagnostic tests and treatments that would be done on and for Quincy. She went through what changes were going to be made in his medications. She told Judy that he needed hospitalization and more aggressive treatment. Their first steps would be radiographs of his lungs and blood work and depending on those results, other steps would be taken.

"Okay, we're going to get him down to radiology, and since we know we're going to keep him for awhile, you can wait for the results in our waiting area or head on back to West Tennessee. We'll call you when we find out something, Mrs. Taylor. Which one would you prefer?" asked Julia.

"You said your name was Dr. Summers, correct?" Judy asked.

"Yes, ma'am, I'm Dr. Summers, and I'm the resident on this rotation." Julia replied.

"Well, no harm intended, but I didn't come here to see you, Dr. Summers, and I didn't come here to see Sara. I came here so a Dr. Sneed could look at Quincy, and I'll be here until he does. If that means that I will be in this exam room or in the waiting area all day, then I'll be here. I hauled him in this shape a long way to see this Dr. Sneed, and I'm not leaving until I see him examine my horse."

Judy was serious, too. She had been patient for close to an hour now, and her patience was running thin. She understood she was at a teaching hospital. She understood Sara had to look at him, and then Dr. Summers had to look at him.

She liked both of these women and to her, they had seemed very competent and caring, but she hadn't come all this way for them. Somewhere, deep in her gut, Judy knew that if she didn't take a stand now, today, Dr. Sneed would never look at her horse.

Sara glanced at Dr. Summers to see her reaction. She had known Mrs. Taylor wouldn't budge, and Dr. Summers might as well get on the phone and call or Judy Taylor would be camping in the exam room. Good for her, thought Sara. She's not afraid of Dr. Sneed or intimidated by his position. He's going to have to step off his pedestal and actually look at a horse. Sara silently cheered for Judy.

"Well, Mrs. Taylor, why don't you let us take Quincy down to radiology and while he's getting his x-rays done, I'll see if I can get in touch with Dr. Sneed?" Julia offered.

"That's fine with me, but I won't leave until he takes a look at Quincy, understand?" Judy retorted.

"Yes, ma'am, we understand. If it's okay with you, though, I'm just going to send Sara on while I get in touch with Dr. Sneed, okay?" Julia asked Judy.

"That'll be fine. I'll be right here - waiting." Judy replied.

"On your way, Sara." Julia instructed Sara.

"Yes, Ma'am." Sara left the room with Quincy in tow and Dr. Summers following behind.

As they exited the exam room with Quincy, Sara could barely repress a smile. She dreaded being in the presence of Dr. Sneed, but more than that, she enjoyed the fact that someone was ordering him around instead of vice versa. He was basically treated as a god and this would be a hard pill for his ego to swallow.

"I thought that was how it would go, Dr. Summers." Sara said shyly.

"I just hope we can get in touch with him. You go ahead and get radiology to do several chest films on this guy. Take some sedation. Get the blood work, too, and turn it into the lab, and I'll work on Dr. Sneed."

"We're on our way." Sara replied as she led Quincy down to a work station to pick up the blood tubes and sedation, draw his blood, and get all the orders in the computer. It wasn't a long walk, but Quincy wasn't doing well. Sara sure wished one of the other students would pass by so she could get some help, and then she saw Hillary.

"Hey, Hillary, can you give me a hand?" Sara called to her classmate.

"Sure, Sara. Looks like you got a lot of work following behind you there. What do you need me to do?"

"I've got to draw blood, get in orders, go to radiology and take the blood down to the lab. If you could run the blood to the lab while I go to radiology, that would be great."

"Sure, Sara. I'll hold him while you get everything in the computer and draw the blood. Then I'll run the blood to the lab. Sound good?"

"Sounds great."

Sara knew she could count on Hillary. She and Hillary were the only two students on the rotation that cared about equine medicine. They volunteered for more cases, worked longer hours, helped each other out and depended on each other. It's not that Sara didn't like her other classmates on the rotation or that they were lazy. Most just figured they would never touch a horse or cow again after vet school. They took their assigned cases, did their jobs, and counted the days until they would be back in the small animal clinic.

With Sara and Hillary, it was different. They couldn't get enough of the large animal clinic and because of their shared interest and large patient load; they had come to rely on each other.

Sara got the orders in the computer and then easily drew Quincy's blood. He never flinched, as most horses would. Sara thought as much. With the full blood tubes in her hand, she looked up at her patient and began stroking his neck. Quincy's large nostrils were flaring wide with each breath. Sweat streamed down his back and neck with his enormous effort to breath. His eyes were frightened and this new place was foreign and scary. The pleading in his eyes was stronger than it had been in the exam room.

He was away from Judy. He was not familiar with his surroundings and the sights and smells of this place seemed to signal possible danger. Sara could tell that even though he was a rational, intelligent horse, he was becoming more stressed by the minute, so she spoke to him in a soothing tone trying to calm him.

"It's okay, big fella', they'll get to us in a minute. You don't have anything to worry about. I know this isn't home and a lot's going on, but you're going to be fine. Just bear with me and we'll have these x-rays done and get you in a stall to make you comfortable. Everything's going to be okay. Just stay calm, and me and you'll have an easy time with it today." Sara cooed to Quincy.

"He's pretty stressed, Sara. I'll take the blood to the lab, but I'm going to run by radiology first to let them know y'all are coming and that he seems critical. You and him take your time getting there and yell out if you need any help, okay?" Hillary asked.

"Sure, and thanks for your help." Sara meant it.

"No problem." Hillary started down the hall and then stopped and turned back to Sara. "You look really tired, you know. You okay?" Hillary asked with genuine concern.

"I'm fine, Hillary. I am tired, but I'm worried. This boy has a lot of sense, and I like him. I just hope we can help him."

Hillary understood and nodded to Sara. "I know, Sara, and whether we like Dr. Sneed or not, you know that if this horse can be helped, he's the one to do it. Have faith, my friend." Hillary turned and continued her journey down the hall.

Chapter 6

Sara led Quincy to radiology. They were ready when she got there. Seth, one of Sara's classmates on the radiology rotation, took Quincy's lead rope and started to lead him into the room. Quincy wouldn't budge. Dusty, another classmate got behind Quincy and started clucking to him and waving his arms trying to coax him forward. Quincy still wouldn't move. He turned and looked at Sara with questioning eyes.

Sara understood why Quincy was hesitant. The large animal x-ray room was located down a long hall with a padded floor. The machines in the room looked like space lasers that moved and rotated on their own. Her classmates were robed in heavy lead aprons for their protection. They looked like butchers from another planet. If Sara hadn't known what all this stuff was and what it was for, she would have been scared, too.

"Hold on a minute, guys. Let me see what I can do." Sara walked back to Quincy, took his lead rope away from Seth and looked into his eyes. "Come on fella', this won't take long and it won't hurt at all, promise. Just trust me." Every step Sara took, Quincy followed and soon, both she and Quincy were standing in the large animal x-ray room.

"Okay, guys, I think y'all can take it from here." Sara handed the lead rope back to Seth and began to walk out.

"Whoa, fella', whoa!" Sara heard Seth yelling behind her. She stopped when she felt a chin on her shoulder and felt Quincy's hard exhalations in her ear. As far as Quincy was concerned, if Sara wasn't staying, he wasn't either. Sara turned to see Seth pulling on Quincy's lead rope while giving her an apologetic grin.

"Guess you're going to have to suit up and stay with us, Sara. Unless you want to give this big boy a lot of drugs, I don't think he's planning on staying in here without you. Dusty will get you an apron." Seth said as he gestured to Dusty to get one of the lead aprons in the corner.

"Okay, guys, let's get this over with." Sara said as Seth handed her the apron, and she slid the monstrous thing on. "Dr. Summers wants several views and as y'all can see from his breathing, I think we'll have plenty to look at when we get these developed."

Dr. Thomas, the radiologist, smiled at Sara as he walked in. He had been her clinician on both of her radiology rotations, and Sara thought the world of him. He was patient, kind, and knowledgeable. He expected you to do well or he wouldn't pass you and you almost had to be flawless to get an A, but he was fair. Sara couldn't ask for a better teacher, and thankfully, most of her professors in this clinical year had been much like Dr. Thomas except, of course, for the present one, Dr. Sneed.

"Hey, Sara, looks like we have an uncooperative patient today. Did you bring some good drugs with you?" Dr. Thomas asked.

"Yeah, I've got them, but I really don't think we'll need them. I just don't think he likes Seth and Dusty, but if you let me stay in here, I think we can get it done, Dr. Thomas." Sara said with a smile while ribbing her classmates.

"Okay, Sara, you take care of our patient and Seth, Dusty, and I will see what kind of pictures we can get you."

For twenty minutes, Sara stroked Quincy's neck and the pair stood motionless as Seth and Dusty took x-rays. Quincy didn't move as long as Sara stayed by his side. Dr. Thomas had given Seth and Dusty orders and then returned behind the scenes to read other x-rays while the guys did their job.

The guys got all their pictures and exited the room to consult with Dr. Thomas. It didn't take them long to come back as Sara and Quincy patiently waited.

"Some weren't up to Thomas's approval, Sara." Seth returned with a sheepish grin.

They went to work again, always making sure both they and Sara were out of the dangerous beam of the x-ray, but still getting good pictures. That's the way it went in the radiology rotation and basically every other rotation during this year. You did it until you got it right - period, and that's the way it should be. As Sara stood with Quincy, she started thinking about the last ten months she had been down at the clinics and all the classroom work before that.

Chapter 7

They called it "down at the clinics" because the clinical portion of the teaching hospital was located on the bottom floor of the veterinary college. Classrooms, labs, libraries, offices, and break rooms were located on the upper floors. Sara had spent three hard years in those classrooms and labs with Seth, Dusty, Hillary, and fifty-five or so more of her classmates. Most of them had made it to clinical rotations, some of them hadn't, and it hadn't gotten any easier once they had made it to the bottom floor.

To become a veterinarian, one had to complete twelve clinical rotations, each lasting a month, and that was after three years of classroom study. Everyone that had made it was in the tenth of twelve rotations, and they had all seen and learned a lot by now.

Over the nearly four years they had been at Knoxville, they had become a rather large family. They knew that you had to work together to achieve your goals even if at times, there was fierce competition between them. The family could be dysfunctional, but when push came to shove, they were there for each other. They had to be. Veterinary students didn't have time for anyone or anything else.

Sara's "brother", Seth, stuck his head back in the room to let her know they were done and the second round of x-rays had satisfied Dr. Thomas's scrutinizing eyes. Sara had been so lost in her own thoughts that she hadn't even realized they had left and were through.

"He said he'd give you the final word in about an hour, Sara. We've got x-rays coming out our ears we've been so busy, so it's going to take awhile."

"Seth, I know you and Dusty have already looked at them. What do you think? How do the big boy's lungs look?" Sara asked already knowing the answer.

"Not good, Sara. I'll come down myself and let you know what Dr. Thomas thinks as soon as he looks at them. Will that be okay?"

"Sure, Seth. You know where I'll be, and thanks."

Sara led Quincy from the radiology department, down the hall, and back into the exam room to Judy Taylor.

"Mrs. Taylor, we've got the x-rays and the bloodwork. I'm going to find Dr. Summers and hopefully, she will have found Dr. Sneed. I'll be right back." Sara turned to go find Dr. Summers and felt Judy Taylor's hand on her arm.

"Wait a minute, Sara, did you get a look at the x-rays?"

"No, ma'am, I didn't, but we should know something soon." Sara knew this woman wanted some good news. She wished she could give Judy some type of hope, but that wasn't her place.

"Thanks. I didn't mean to hold you up."

"No problem, Mrs. Taylor. Ask me anything anytime. I'm going to go on and see if I can find Dr. Summers, okay?"

"Sure, Sara, I'll be right here."

Sara found Dr. Summers waiting down the hall. "He'll be down in a minute. You get everything else done?"

"Yes ma'am. I guess we are just all waiting for him now. I hope he comes soon."

And, for once, he did.

Chapter 8

Dr. Timothy Sneed burst through the double doors with both an annoyed and questioning look on his face. He had been pulled away from important research data in his office to see a persistent client and was not in the least bit happy about the situation. Sara even had to admit that even though she disliked the man, he did look much more professional than either she or Dr. Summers.

With his long, white lab coat, khaki pants, button up shirt, and tie, he immediately demanded respect. Dr. Sneed was not a handsome man, but his tall, lanky presence and his determined stride did set him apart. Sara thought that it could have been possible for this graying dark-haired man with the determined jaw to be handsome if it weren't for his long, crooked nose and those beady, dark eyes so aptly covered with small, round-rimmed framed glasses. Sara had sneaked a glance into those eyes only once, and what she had seen there was a clinical machine with no regard or compassion for either patients or students. This quality, too, added to his unfavorable appearance.

"Where is she?" he demanded.

"First exam room." Julia replied.

He continued his stride down the hall until he entered the exam room. There, upon seeing Judy Taylor, all annoyance faded from his face and a forced grin appeared upon his lips. He held out his hand to Judy Taylor with practiced ease.

"Hello, Mrs. Taylor, I'm Dr. Sneed. Dr. Summers tells me that you have a pretty sick guy here." He spoke to Judy as if he had known her all her life and had quickly changed from the bothered genius to the helpful and sincere veterinarian down the street. Sara thought she might vomit.

"Hello, Dr. Sneed. Quincy and I have been waiting for you, and we're glad to see you. Can you see what you can do for my boy?" Judy had brightened the moment Dr. Sneed had entered the room.

"Sure, let's see what we have here." Dr. Sneed replied. Timothy Sneed quickly looked through Quincy's history and, again, Quincy was given a physical exam. Sara set back and watched the master hoping fervently that neither she nor Dr. Summers had left anything out.

When Dr. Sneed finished his physical and looked at the tests she and Dr. Summers had already ordered, he turned to Julia and asked if they had any results. Julia turned to Sara.

"No, sir, not yet. Radiology is supposed to let me know something within the hour. " Sara replied.

Without acknowledging that Sara had ever spoken, Dr. Sneed basically reiterated what Dr. Summers had already told Judy. They would wait for the test results and possibly, do more testing. They would probably change the medication. They would have to see what radiology said, and finally, Quincy would have to stay here until he was stable.

"Will Sara be taking care of him under your supervision, Dr. Sneed?" Judy Taylor asked.

"Sara?" Dr. Sneed threw a questioning glance at Dr. Summers. She quickly glanced over to Sara to let him know that the student did indeed have a name. Sara caught it all, but thankfully, Judy Taylor did not.

"Oh, of course Mrs. Taylor, if that's what you would like. Sara can keep you apprised of things." Dr. Sneed replied.

"That'll be fine," Judy said. "Now, if y'all don't mind, I'd like to have just a couple of minutes alone with Quincy before I head back home.

"Of course, Mrs. Taylor. Just let the student, uh, I mean Sara, know when you're done." And with that, Dr. Sneed set down Quincy's record and motioned for Dr. Summers and Sara to follow him out of the room leaving Judy and Quincy alone.

Judy stood with Quincy by her side, and for a minute, she couldn't find her voice. Her companion and friend for all these years at once understood, and with great effort brought his head down to her knee and began sliding it up to her shoulder. He rested his head on her shoulder and let out a deep sigh.

As tears ran down her cheeks, Judy spoke to Quincy for what she thought might be the last time.

"I love you, fella'. Always have, always will. You know I wouldn't leave you if I didn't think they could fix you. I'm sorry I had to put you through this morning with you feelin' this bad, but you understand, don't you? I think that little girl will take care of you, buddy. I really think she will, and the doctors here, they'll treat you right. I can't stay here with you, but I'll be back to get you, fella, one way or the other. I'll be back for you. Get better for me, okay?"

Judy gave Quincy a kiss on the noise to say goodbye and, with a determination she did not feel, called Sara back into the room. Dr. Sneed and Julia stayed in the hall.

"Sara, take good care of him for me, okay? Stay in touch with me and let me know what's happening up here. I expect at least one or two calls from you a day, and I always want you to be honest with me and do what's best for him. No matter what, you promise me?"

"Yes, ma'am. I promise. I'll call you every day and let you know how he's doing."

"And you'll be honest, yes?"

"Yes, ma'am, I promise."

"Even if it's time to let him go, you'll tell me straight, right, Sara? Don't let him suffer."

"Yes, even then, Mrs. Taylor. I won't let him suffer."

"Okay, then, I'm leaving my boy in your hands, and Sara, I'm trusting you. Do you hear me? I'm going to trust you." Judy looked deep into Sara's eyes and Sara knew she meant what she was saying. "Do NOT let him suffer, if y'all can't fix him."

"Yes, ma'am, Mrs. Taylor."

"Okay, I'm going to finish things up here in the office and be on my way. He's yours now."

Judy handed the lead rope to Sara, gave Quincy a big hug, and left the room. Quincy followed Judy with his eyes until she left the room and then turned his attention back to Sara as if to say, "Alright, you heard her. Take care of me. I want to feel better."

Chapter 9

Sara led Quincy out into the hall where Dr. Sneed and Dr. Summers were discussing his case. Seth had personally handed the radiology report to Dr. Summers, and the lab reports were in. Quincy's lungs and his blood work showed pneumonia along with his primary problem, COPD. A preliminary regimen of IV fluids and antibiotics were agreed upon as well as medications to help his breathing.

If they saw no improvement quickly, other tests for Quincy would be ordered to determine the exact cause for his pneumonia as well as how best to deal with it. When all was said and done, Sara would be treating Quincy with antibiotics and inhalers four times daily, every six hours, around the clock.

"I expect you to have his medications picked up at the pharmacy, have him in his stall, on IV fluids, and comfortable plus all the paperwork done by 2pm today to start his breathing treatment and IV antibiotics, Sara. If you wait and do the breathing treatment and IV antibiotics at two o'clock, it will have you and him on a better schedule. Get Stephanie to help you, if she's got the time. If not, find a way to get it done. Any questions?" Dr. Summers asked as she and Dr. Sneed turned to exit the large animal clinic.

"No, ma'am." Sara replied. It was now eleven o'clock. That gave her three hours before Quincy's breathing treatment. All she had to do was call Stephanie, get Quincy bedded down in his stall, hooked up to IV fluids, pick up his meds at the pharmacy, and administer some lunch-time treatments to a few of her other patients. If she could get in touch with Stephanie, she should have time to grab some lunch and go to the library before two o'clock.

Sara led Quincy to his designated stall and got him settled in. Now, she just had all the other things to do for him and treat her other patients. As Sara walked to the closest phone and picked up the receiver, Stephanie, one of the large animal vet techs, appeared like a ghost from one of the exam room doors.

"Boy, I'm glad you're here. Dr. Summers said to get you if I could, but I didn't know what your schedule would be today."

"Happy to help, Sara. I saw Dr. Summers in the hall, and she filled me in on what needs to be done. Don't let her fool you, she may have told you to do this all by yourself, but she was out in the hall looking for me. She knows you need some help especially with the other patients you have and the night you had last night. What do you want to do first?"

"I guess get his IV started and get his paperwork done. I'll go by and pick up his meds on my way to lunch. Sound like a plan to you?"

"Let's get started."

It took a little over an hour for Sara and Stephanie to get everything done. Alone, it would have taken Sara much longer, but Stephanie was wonderful. Sara respected her talents and her knowledge. Unlike some of her classmates, Sara was not threatened by Stephanie's skills. Sara knew that it wasn't just the professors and the residents that could teach her something, but all the vet techs, like Stephanie, were a wealth of information. Sara didn't mind taking full advantage of their knowledge.

When all was said and done, Quincy looked pretty comfortable in his stall. Sara smiled as he stuck his head out of the stall to look at his new surroundings.

"At least he's still interested in what's going on. Maybe we have a chance, Steph."

"He looks bad, Sara, but he may have some hope. They can work miracles here."

"I know. That's what me and Hillary were talking about earlier. I just hope they have one for him."

"You never know, Sara. The great veterinary practitioner in the sky decides who will go and who will stay, but I'm like you, I hope we have one left for him."

Stephanie and Sara stood there, in silence, for a brief moment at the front of Quincy's stall, watching him struggle to breathe but somehow finding the strength to fight on. The four five liter IV bags hung from a special hook attached to the ceiling of the stall. The clear IV tubing attached to the ports in the lower bags and ran down in a spiral snake that coiled and uncoiled with Quincy's movement, so he would not be inhibited as he moved around the stall. The IV catheter, which measured two inches long, was now safely inside the jugular vein in Quincy's neck with the hub of the catheter super-glued to his neck and fastened securely with sutures to his skin. Only the hub of the catheter shown as it met with the tubing to deliver much needed fluids, and soon, medicine to its patient.

They had put special bedding in his stall to decrease allergens that might aggravate his condition. They had also made small adjustments in his diet to decrease dust and allergens, and in a couple of hours, Sara would have to place a mask on his nose and give him breathing treatments. Quincy, she knew, would do fine.

Most horses would have balked at the IV catheter placement and all the tubes and strange surroundings. Quincy had not. He had stood stoically as Sara and Stephanie had inserted the catheter, hooked him to the tubing and placed the sutures into the skin of his neck. Sara was pretty sure he would be good for the breathing treatment, too. He was just that kind of horse - he knew they were trying to help.

"Well, Sara, I'll say a little prayer for your guy, and if you need anything else, I'm here. You got it covered for now?"

"Yeah, Steph, I think I can handle it from here. I've got a couple of other patients to treat, and then I'm going to try and get some lunch. Thanks for all your help. I really appreciate it."

"No, problem. Any time. All you got to do is call me. Let me know how he does, Sara. I'll be thinking about you. But, right now, I've got other fish to fry and more students to help. See you later."

Stephanie left just as she had come, like a vapor that moves silently through the halls of the large animal clinic appearing just in time to help a student through a procedure, hook up an IV, or administer medication. Sara was sure she would see her again when it was time to treat Quincy. Stephanie would stand back, in the corner, making sure no help was needed and everything was going okay.

As Sara turned back to Quincy, she couldn't help the little laugh that escaped from her lips. Even though he was very sick, Quincy looked better and more relaxed in the stall that he had earlier in the exam room or radiology department. He had actually decided to eat a little and had stopped his munching long enough to acknowledge Stephanie's departure and was now looking at Sara with a quizzical expression.

"Everything good, Buddy, cause if it is, I'll just tell you, I've got other patients besides you, and I'm starving. You think it would be okay for me to go get some lunch and treat my other patients? I know you think you're special, but in case you haven't noticed, you're not the only one here."

Quincy turned and looked at Sara as if to say everything was good, and even though he thought he was the only important patient here, it was okay for her to treat the others and get some lunch. This plush stall was pretty neat, and the feed tasted quite good. The IV fluids were already making him feel better, and he would just wait right here until his breathing treatment in the afternoon. He wasn't nervous anymore, and she could go ahead and do whatever else needed to be done.

"Okay then, Quincy, I'm off, and I'll see you in about two hours, Big Boy. Be good while I'm gone and try to feel better."

Chapter 10

With his slight improvement in such a short time and his spunky attitude, there was definitely a chance. By the time Sara had finished treating her other patients and made her way to the break room for lunch, she found herself thinking that Quincy just might be fine. All her other patients were rapidly improving, so Quincy should be okay, too. After all, he had one of the premiere equine specialist in the country looking out for him, a resident that was an extremely bright, compassionate workaholic, and Sara who had already made up her mind that this guy was going to live.

As Sara placed her worn dollar in the coke machine to purchase a diet coke, a couple of second and third year students in the break room waved and looked her way in recognition. She knew their faces, but sadly, she couldn't really remember their names. They were all dressed in their nice classroom clothes, and Sara knew she looked like a vagabond from the street with her unruly hair, wrinkled coveralls, and deep bags under her eyes. She didn't care, though. Even though she liked most of the underclassmen, she didn't know them well, and they had no idea what was waiting for them when they entered their clinical year.

The first three years had been hard and there were plenty of sleepless nights studying for tests and memorizing thousands of pages of material dealing with physiology, anatomy, cardiology, radiology, and the list went on and on, but when you went to clinics, it all came together, and you better be able to perform. Clinics probably didn't demand more time than the first three years when you were in class from eight to five every day, went home, got some dinner, and then studied late into the night. But in clinics, the cases weren't just data and statistics on a page. They were real breathing, living animals like Quincy who needed your help, and that made all the difference.

Sara looked at these underclassmen and was glad she was now through those years. Yes, clinics were for real, and it was hard and more responsibility, but you actually did get to see what all your years of hard work could accomplish. Of course, the interns, residents, and clinicians kept a close eye on the fourth year students, but as the clinical year had advanced, the tight rein these supervisors held on the students became looser to allow fourth years students to realize what it felt like to practice veterinary medicine.

With Quincy's case, Sara was glad those specialist still held those reins, even if loosely. She knew she would do most of the work on his case, but she would still have the knowledge and advice of Dr. Summers and if needed, Dr. Sneed. She wouldn't be working this difficult case alone, but in a few short months, whatever case she saw would be her sole responsibility, and even with the confidence she had gained, that thought was intimidating. Too intimidating to think about right now and right here.

The break room was noisy and too many people were around. Sara needed some time to herself to think about nothing and to find some quiet. She decided to go to the courtyard.

The weather was still a little cool this time of year, so Sara knew there wouldn't be many students in the courtyard outside the library. She took her diet coke and a package of peanut butter and crackers she had also purchased from the vending machine and headed outside to get some fresh air.

The courtyard was completely empty, as Sara had hoped. It was a good place to sit and relax. The courtyard was a quiet place nestled between the library and the classroom portion of the veterinary school with the Cumberland River in view across the street. Trees and flowers of all kinds dotted the little hiding place, and in just a few more weeks, most would be in bloom. Sara had rested here many times before, and as she watched the waves of the river silently sway to the spring breeze, she began to relax.

Chapter 11

As Sara's eyes began to close, and her head nod forward, Sara pictured the river at home in her mind. This was early to be fishing on the river, but her Daddy and she would have probably given it a try on a day like this anyway.

They'd get up early, get ready, and leave in the misty haze of morning just when the moon was falling behind the trees and the sun was beginning to rise. There was a little diner on the way where they would stop for breakfast, drink coffee, and talk. Just a few miles down, the gravel country road would veer sharply down and into the Tennessee River where they would unload the boat into the water.

The morning would still be cool by the time they got on the river. The motor would cut through the silence of the morning as they took off to their favorite fishing hole, and Sara would gaze at the morning sky as it met the blue-green waters of the river. They would cut the motor off a couple of minutes before they got to their fishing hole and start the trolling motor so all the fish wouldn't be scared away.

Sara would cast her line into the water and watch as the red and white bobber lulled back and forth with the flow of the river.

"What's that up there on the bank, Baby?" her Daddy would ask.

"Is that a horse, Daddy? Has someone left their horse here on the river bank?"

"Sara, he looks like he's not feeling very good. Aren't you supposed to be taking care of him? Wake up now, Honey, you got work to do. I know you're tired, but wake up. He looks like he needs you."

As her Daddy was urging Sara to wake up, the horse on the bank turned to look at Sara, and then, it spoke.

"Sara, you need to wake up and go to the pharmacy and get my afternoon medications. You know I need them and here you are out fishing with your Daddy. You probably need to go by the library, too. Wake up or I'll tell Dr. Sneed and Judy about you." The dream horse said.

Sara lurched awake and checked her watch almost simultaneously. She had only been napping about fifteen minutes; just long enough to let the chill from the concrete bench find its way through the thin, crummy overalls and numb her legs and rear end. She shook her head, grinned sideways and rolled her eyes at the dream. It would be nice to stay out here and just enjoy the breeze and the river, but as the dream had so pointedly reminded her, it was time to get back to work.

Sara stopped in the library and plunked down at a computer to gather more facts about Quincy's disease. Once she got home tonight, if she ever got home, she would bring out the textbooks and the notes, but right now, she needed the accuracy and the speed that could only be found on the Internet.

Sara put her search words in one of her favorite sites, and when thousands of hits came back, she scanned down to sources that she knew were reliable. She had seen so many horse owners come in believing everything they read on the Internet that she knew and had been taught not to make the same mistake. They would crucify you in clinics if you started quoting some of the crap those sites guaranteed were facts. Sara started with the veterinary journals and went from there.

An hour later with notes jotted down in her handy-dandy pocket notebook and hundreds of facts in her head, Sara headed down to the pharmacy. She still had thirty minutes until Quincy's two o'clock treatment, and she should be right on schedule.

The line at the pharmacy was short, but Sara had a lot of meds to pick up plus the mask for Quincy that would deliver his medication. When she finished at the pharmacy, she had ten minutes to be back down to his stall.

When she arrived at Quincy's stall five minutes before two, Dr. Summers and the rest of the students on the rotation, including Hillary, were waiting for her. Stephanie was at the workstation looking busy, but Sara was pretty sure she wasn't doing a thing except making sure Sara wouldn't need any help.

"Cut it kinda' close, didn't you, Sara?" curtly asked Dr. Summers.

"Yes, Dr. Summers, but I have everything here and ready. Do you want me to go ahead and treat him or had you rather do it the first time?" asked Sara.

"You go ahead, Sara, and if you have any trouble, just let me know. We'll all be watching." Dr. Summers replied.

"Okay, then. Here we go." Sara sighed.

Chapter 12

Sara put Quincy's halter on, attached the lead rope, and gave the big guy a pleading look to be good with so many watching. The intravenous injections Sara had to give Quincy were a snap. He already had a port in his fluid line where she could inject without re-sticking him and causing him any pain.

It was the breathing treatment Sara was worried about. She hoped she could figure how to get the mask on his head and the canister on the mask to deliver his medicine, so it could deliver its mist of pharmaceuticals that would expand his bronchi and help him to breathe. Sara hesitated looking at the contraption, and as almost on cue, Hillary slid inside the stall.

"Need me to hold him for you while you get that together?" Hillary asked.

"Sure, that would be great." Sara replied gratefully.

Thank God for friends. Sara knew she should have already had one or two practice runs putting the mask on Quincy before the whole crew showed up, but she had assumed she would be treating him alone with Dr. Summers showing up after Sara had figured it out. Well, that's what assuming got you.

Sara knew from the pictures she had seen while in the library on the internet that the strap fit over his ears and the clear looking portion with all the funny parts fit over his muzzle. If she could just figure out which port the canister with the medications fit in, she would be good to go.

As Sara was puzzling over how to get the thing together, she heard a soft, broken whinny coming from her stall mate, and it wasn't Hillary. Quincy could tell she was nervous, and in his way, was letting her know to slow down and calm down and everything would be okay. He would be a good boy and do anything she asked. She just needed to take a breath and get everything together.

Like magic, the canister seemed to roll to a port where only it would fit, and as she went to place the strap over his ears and the clear portion of the mask with all its ports over his nose, she could have sworn Quincy winked at her. Sara placed the canister in the correct port and blew a puff of much needed medication in the mask for Quincy to breathe.

He didn't wince, snort, move, and as far as Sara could see, blink, except for the supposed wink through it all. He was, in all accounts, the perfect patient. Sara took in a deep breath and sighed with relief.

"Looks good, Sara. Now when you are through with the inhaler, come on out here and tell us all what you know about COPD that you didn't know this morning, what were the medications you just gave him and how they work, and if and when you will order other tests to further investigate your patient's problem." Dr. Summers never missed a beat.

So, when Sara finished with Quincy's treatment and removed the mask from his face, she stepped outside the stall and with her classmates, went over Quincy's case, his disease, its causes, treatments, and further testing that might be needed. Dr. Summers asked a couple of questions, her classmates asked a couple of questions, and thankfully, in the end, Sara answered them all.

"Okay, guys, time to go back to work. Everybody has his or her patients to attend to and new patients coming in. I'll see you all in late afternoon rounds." Julia Summers paused, "Let's get to it, and Sara, hold on a minute, I want to talk to you before you go." Dr. Summers watched as all the other students in the rotation left to get back to the day's business and then she turned to Sara.

"Jessica is on emergency tonight, so she'll take care of Quincy's treatments tonight. Your other patients are either ready to go home or don't need treatment until the morning. Hillary and Josh have volunteered to take some of your incoming afternoon patients. If any need hospitalization, you will need to take over tomorrow morning. They also said they could fill you in tomorrow on today's afternoon rounds.

By the time you work up the discharge instructions for your patients that are going home and talk with their owners, you will have been here going on thirty-six hours, and if you stay to treat Quincy for his eight o'clock, that'll be close to forty. After you finish talking to your clients and get their animals on the way home, you go home and get some rest."

Dr. Summers continued, "I wouldn't usually do this, but we don't know how long Quincy will be with us. While he is with us, you will get very limited sleep because of his treatment schedule and your clinic schedule. Take tonight and be back here in the morning. Don't argue with me - this is a one time favor."

Julia didn't wait for Sara to protest, as she knew she would. She simply turned around and walked down the hall to check on patients and her students. Julia did not know if Sara had thought about the fact that she would be treating Quincy every six hours after today, but Julia had, and with other patients coming in all the time, Julia knew Sara needed at least one good night's rest before the ordeal really began.

Sara's classmates would help her today and tonight, but tomorrow, Quincy would be solely Sara's responsibility. The rotation still had one more week, and if the horse lasted that long, Sara could be looking at a very long, sleepless week. Sleep deprivation was normal in this profession, and Julia wanted to teach them that, but even veterinarians in practice had help every once in awhile. Julia wanted to teach them that, too.

Julia wondered if Sara would hold up to the strain, but then she remembered the way Sara had looked at Quincy and wonders of wonders, how that horse had nickered at Sara when she had fumbled with his meds. He had even winked at her. There was something between those two, and Julia knew what it was. She had also felt it with some of her patients.

Sara would give Quincy her all, of that, Julia was sure.

Sara stood at the stall watching Julia disappear. She had barely comprehended Dr. Summer's words. Sleep? Go home? Let someone else treat your patient? Sara thought she must really look tired because she had not heard those words from Julia Summers before, but she wasn't going to question them.

The fifteen minute power nap back at the court yard had revived her a little, but now that fuzzy, icky feeling of exhaustion was beginning to creep back up on her again, and sleep was what

Sara wanted most in the world - peaceful, glorious sleep, but then Sara remembered her patient.

"You going to be okay if I leave, fella'?" Sara asked Quincy, and as if to reassure her, he stuck his head outside the stall and gave her shoulder a small, little push. Sara knew it was only her hopeful mind that saw him breathing with a little less effort and his eyes letting her know he was maybe a tiny bit more comfortable, but that push was all she needed.

"I'm going to go and get some of my other patients ready to go home, and just think, maybe in a week or so, I might be getting discharge papers ready for you, Boy, wouldn't that be wonderful?" Sara asked Quincy.

As if in response, Quincy's head bobbed up and down ever so slightly.

"Okay, I'll see you in the morning. I bet you'll be feeling better by then, fella'." With one last pat to Quincy's head, Sara headed to the office to get everything together for her other patients.

It took Sara about an hour to get her patients discharged and talk with their owners. She talked with the owners extensively about the animal's care when it went home and what to look for if they needed to bring the animal back or call. Sara was pretty confident with the health of the patients she sent home, and when she had discharged the last one, she closed the chart, went to the women's locker room to change clothes, picked her purse up as she was walking out the door, and finally, climbed in her pickup.

Chapter 13

The traffic on Neyland Drive wasn't bad this afternoon, and even downtown, it wasn't crowded. She turned on Chapman Highway, and before she knew it, was pulling up at her apartment complex. Sara had chosen to live alone this last year of vet school. She had classmates as her roommates up until this year, but it seemed as if everyone was getting ready to go their own way during the clinical year, and that was fine with Sara.

It had been wonderful to live and study with classmates the first couple of years, but in clinics, somehow it was different. Your downtime was your alone time, and it was hard to be alone in an apartment with roommates.

Leanne, one of Sara's classmates and friends, lived in the same apartment complex, and that was how she had found this inexpensive, yet safe and relatively modern complex. She and Leanne would visit each other depending on their schedules, and they looked out for each other. Sara, however, was too tired for visiting this afternoon. She just wanted some sleep and to be by herself.

By herself, that is, except for the warm body waiting up in her one bedroom apartment whom Sara had not seen since early yesterday morning. As Sara climbed the three flights up to her apartment, she could hardly wait to see her man. She turned the key, opened the door, and there he came bounding out of the bedroom to greet her.

"Wait a minute, now, I'm really tired. You are going to have to calm down a minute." Sara cooed at her roommate.

As he jumped into her arms, she felt his cold, black nose nuzzle her neck and his little pink tongue dart to lick her face, nose, and ears.

"Calm down, Jake. Momma needs some sleep. I know Leanne has been coming up here to walk and play with you. You haven't been alone all this time, so don't even give me this guilt trip."

Jake continued to squirm in her arms and wet her face with his quick, little kisses. Sara had decided to get this blue heeler pup against her better judgment. She knew she didn't need a puppy while in clinics, but Leanne had vowed to help her raise him. The landlord had not been too keen on the idea, but Sara had assured him that if you couldn't trust veterinary students to raise a puppy right, whom could you trust? So, the landlord had agreed.

Sara had paid the pet deposit and immediately driven two hours to pick the little monster up. She remembered the drive home like it was yesterday. The pups coloring with the speckled grey, white and black hairs mottled throughout his coat actually made him look blue. He had a dark, black mask around his left eye that extended all the way to his left ear. His ears were still floppy, now, but one day, they would stand straight up – always in alert.

Sara had chosen him from the litter because he had been the one that had hung back and watched Sara as all the others had rushed to her jumping on her shin with their tiny paws and pulling at her pants leg with their sharp little teeth. Jake had watched, and when his siblings had tired of the visitor, he had cautiously walked up to her, set down in front of her and cocked his head to take a good look.

Sara was sure her love affair with the pup had begun that moment, but if there had been any doubt, the ride home had cemented her affection for him. Jake had sit in the passenger's side as Sara had started her truck and began the drive back to Knoxville. For a total of two minutes, the young pup quietly looked at his surroundings, tried to see out the window, and fidgeted in the passenger's seat. Sara glanced his way, and as she did, he began to whine.

"You already miss your brothers and sisters, buddy?" Sara asked.

Jake had whined louder.

"The ride isn't already making you sick, is it?"

Jake had begun to howl.

"Okay, okay, little one. I shouldn't be doin' this, but see if the ride is easier in my lap."

And, it must have been. For as soon as Sara placed the pup in her lap, he calmed down. He then proceeded to circle her lap with his small stocky legs and plop down for a nap. Sara knew this was a bad way to start the pup. She knew it wasn't a brilliant idea to be riding down the interstate with a puppy in her lap, but he was quiet, and that was going to have to be enough for now.

Jake slept for most of the ride home only waking to peer up at Sara with those sharp brown eyes surrounded by the black mask. She would stroke his fat puppy body occasionally on the ride and try to watch the road while she also watched his steady breathing up and down.

Jake only had one or two puppy dreams on the ride home. The pup's legs would tremble or he would whimper in his dream. Sara would place her hand on him to reassure him, and then she would hear the suckling noise all young make when they are dreaming of their mothers and the security they feel in their presence.

By the time Sara had navigated her way through Knoxville traffic and arrived safely at her apartment, the love affair was sealed. Sara remembered the pup waking up as she turned off her truck, and true to blue heeler form, he had been awake ever since. His energy was boundless, and Sara found herself wondering at times why she had taken on this project so soon before graduating and still in clinics, and then, Jake would look at her or follow her or need her in such a way that all her reservations would vanish. Just like he was doing now.

Jake's ears would straightened from time to time now, and as she held him in her arms, he held both ears at rapt attention and gazed into Sara's eyes. Even though he was still a pup, Sara could see his future grace, his unending loyalty, and his boundless love for her in those eyes. He knew his master was tired. He knew she wouldn't have left him this long unless it was absolutely necessary, and after his initial excitement at seeing her, he began to calm down knowing Sara was not herself.

"It's okay, Jake. Momma just needs some sleep. We'll take you out, and maybe play with the ball for a while to get you wound down, and then I'll go to bed. Come on, let's go outside for a minute."

Jake wiggled from her arms at the mention of outside, and before Sara could get his leash, he was waiting at the door. Back down the steps with the bounding puppy Sara went, and as they finally reached the grass, Jake walked two or three steps, did his business, and then signaled to Sara he was ready to go back in.

"Don't you want to stay out and get some fresh air, Jake?"

The pup pulled at the leash heading back toward the steps and inside. Sara obeyed the pup, and once inside, went to get the ball in the bedroom. Jake followed her in and went to the bed. At first, Sara thought the pup may have been playing with the ball and rolled it under the bed and was letting Sara know where his ball was. Instead, the pup stretched his little body up to put his front paws on the bed.

Sara stood in the bedroom puzzled.

"You don't want to play with the ball either, buddy?"

The pup looked at Sara and whined.

"You ready to go to bed?"

He started jumping on his back legs trying to get into the bed even though it would be at least another month before he would have the height or the strength to make that jump.

"Okay, fella.' Let me put on my pajamas, get my book, and we'll both climb in. Maybe you haven't slept well with me gone."

Sara took only a second to put on her pajamas. She needed to try and read more on COPD, so she also went to her bookcase and pulled an equine internal medicine textbook off the shelf. She walked back to the bed and pulled back the covers.

The crisp, clean sheets looked immensely inviting, and the warm fuzzy comforter held the promise of sweet, comfortable sleep. Sara lifted Jake into the bed, and then she climbed in herself with book in hand. She opened her book to the chapter on respiratory diseases and began to read. After a few minutes, her eyes begin to slowly close.

The last thing she remembered before she fell into blissful sleep was the blue heeler pup. He had situated himself in his place on the bed, the pillow beside her. He was lying on his stomach on top of the pillow.

His blue puppy head with the dark, black mask was between his spotted puppy paws. His ears were alert and his eyelids were not closing in sleep. His sharp, brown eyes were watching Sara, protecting Sara, if needed. She remembered thinking that he hadn't been sleepy at all, but he had known she was exhausted.

What a good little man he was, and with that thought, the darkness began to descend, the book dropped from her hands, and her thoughts gave way to deep, peaceful sleep.

Chapter 14

Sara was awakened by the scream of the telephone on the nightstand. Her first thought was that she had overslept. She checked her clock. It read 2:15 a.m. Who in the world was calling her at this hour and was something wrong? As she jerked up the receiver, she got her answer to both as she heard the voice of her classmate, Jessica.

"Sara, you there? Sara?" Jessica asked.

"Yeah, Jess, I'm here. What's the matter? Is something wrong?" Sara asked in return.

"Quincy won't let me treat him. He did fine with the eight o'clock treatment, but he's really fighting me on this one, and it's wearing him out. Doug is here with me. Between the two of us, we can probably get him treated, but it's going to really stress him." Jessica continued, "I just wanted to let you know in case you wanted to come."

"Give me a minute to get on some clothes, and I'll be down there." Sara was already climbing out of bed and looking for her clothes.

"You sure, Sara?"

"Yeah, I'm sure. Just try and not excite him before I get there."

"Okay. I'll treat some of my other patients while I'm waiting. Just give me a call on my cell when you get here, and I'll help."

"Okay, Jess. I'll see you in about fifteen."

Sara hung up the phone, and looked over to Jake who had finally curled up in a little ball and gone to sleep. The phone had also awakened him, and he stared questioningly at Sara.

"I've got to go back, Jake. You want to take a ride?"

At the word 'ride', Jake snapped to attention. Even though she had only had him a few weeks, he had quite the vocabulary and 'ride' was definitely a word he understood.

"Let's go, fella'."

Sara dressed in no time, but Jake was already sitting at the front door to go on the ride. She snapped his leash on and out they went, down the steps, and into the cool night air. Sara unlocked the truck, took the puppy in her arms, and both settled in the driver's seat which, again, Sara knew was a bad idea, but she just couldn't help herself.

Jake had learned to stay still and quiet as long as he was sitting in Sara's lap, and if she moved him to the passenger's side, he would begin that loud, high pitched howl of his. She wasn't sure what she would do with the puppy when he got to be a fifty-pound dog, but she would worry about that later. Right now, the important thing was to get back to the large animal clinic.

As Sara and Jake drove through the quiet, wooded apartment complex with just a few street lamps burning, she couldn't help but compare the place she had picked to live her last year in Knoxville to home. At home, it always seemed quiet, and the city lights were far away. The only lights in the night sky at home were the bright stars twinkling over the crest of the trees.

Her parents back porch was just a concrete slab, but beyond that porch was a large back yard. At the end of that back yard stood an old wooden barn with a metal roof, and beyond that, soft rolling hills that stopped just short of woods that seemed to go on for miles.

Sara had spent most of her childhood in, around, and outside of that barn. Her father had loved horses, and Sara could never remember being without one. Her first memory was of riding with her father. She could still remember how the grass had raced by far below her as the wind had blown onto her face and through her hair. She had felt as if she was soaring.

The sky had been so blue above her, and she had known, even at the age of three, this must be what it felt like to fly. She could remember that she had not been scared, because she knew she was safe held in the cradle of her daddy's strong arms. She could remember the saddle horn in front of her, her daddy riding in the saddle behind her, and the horse's mane flying in the wind. She had not a care in the world.

Sara found herself wishing for that carefree time again as she pulled into the back parking lot of the clinic. She turned off the motor and willed herself back to the now and Quincy. If Quincy was going to be a problem, she needed to have all her senses about her. Even though he was sick, he was still big with lightening fast reflexes and speed. Sara looked down at the pup in her lap and let out a long, tired sigh.

"Jake, you're going to have to wait here because I'm not sure what's going to be happening in there, and I don't need for you to get stomped tonight with everything else that's going on. I'll crack the windows for you, and see if you can get some more sleep. I've got a little chew bone for you in the dash to occupy your time just in case you get fidgety." The pup listened as Sara gave her instructions.

Sara lugged the pup over to the passenger's side, presented him with the bone which he found of great interest, and cracked the windows on the truck. He was fine on the passenger's side as long as she wasn't in the truck, and he had something to gnaw on.

"Try not to pee in the truck while I'm gone, okay?" Jake just looked at Sara as if to say, "I'm only a puppy, woman. What do you expect?"

Sara climbed out of the truck. As she walked with a determined stride into the clinic, she worried about what she might find once she arrived at Quincy's stall, and when she finally did get there, her worries were confirmed.

Chapter 15

Quincy was streaming wet with sweat and his breathing was rapid and shallow. He was constantly pacing back and forth in his stall, and Sara could see that he was both irritated and excited. She flipped open her cell phone, turned to get his meds from the nearby workstation, and dialed Jessica's number.

"What on earth did y'all do to the guy, Jess?" Sara asked in the calmest voice she could muster.

"Are you here?" Jessica responded.

"Yeah, I'm standing at this stall, and he looks awful!"

"Calm down, Sara, I'll be right there." Jessica hung up without another word.

While Sara had been talking to Jessica, she had been looking on the workstation for Quincy's meds. She found them and then was struck by the silence coming from Quincy's stall. She could still hear the loud, raspy breathing, but to her ears, it seemed the pacing had ceased.

She turned her head to look over at the stall, and saw Quincy looking out at her. It almost looked as if the horse was saying, "I don't trust anyone else but you. You are going to treat me, and I'll be a good boy for you. Understand? Now, get over here and give me some relief."

"So, this is how it's going to be, huh?" She questioned the horse, and she could almost swear by the look in his eyes and the tilt of his head that he answered her with, "Yeah, this is how it's going to be."

About that time, Jessica rounded the corner in a rush. Doug was with her. That was interesting - Doug wasn't on emergency. Both stopped cold when they saw Sara and the horse and began to smile.

"I can't believe it, Sara. This is the easiest I've seen him all night. I hate you had to come, but it's a relief that he's finally calmed down." Jessica said.

"Don't worry about it, Jess. I'm going to treat him from now on. I don't think he'll fight me, but if you don't mind, just stay for a minute so we can see what he does, okay?"

"Sure, Sara. I'll be waiting right here."

Sara went into the stall. Quincy stood there. He did not pace; he did not try to move; he did not try to escape to the far end of the stall. He just stood there as Sara treated him.

As the IV drip and inhaler delivered the medications that would hopefully make Quincy better, Sara stood there and stroked his long neck being careful not to dislodge the catheter or the IV line. Through it all, he was a trooper, and when Sara had finished, she collected her syringes and stepped out of the stall.

"Well, that went much better than I had expected." Jessica told Sara.

"I think he's just that kind of horse that only trusts one or two people, and I'm one of them. Don't take it to heart, Jess. He just doesn't know you."

"Sara, he really doesn't know you either, but he let you do whatever you needed to do. You have a way with him, and that's just it. If you want me to, I'll treat him for you in the morning, so you can get some more sleep, but, honestly, if I was you- I'd be here."

"Don't worry. I will be. If you have any trouble from him tonight, just call me. I can be here in just a couple of minutes."

"As long as I don't have to treat him, I don't think we'll have any problems. I just hate you had to come back and do it."

"But, that's my job, isn't it, Jess?"

"Yeah, Sara, that's your job, but I'll help anytime I can."

Jessica smiled at Sara, and Sara smiled back knowing Jessica would help if needed. They were all a team here.

"Thanks, Jessica. Doug, you've been awfully quiet. What are you doing here tonight?" Sara redirected.

"Oh, thought I'd just come down to see what was going on tonight." Doug replied.

"Really? I don't usually make it down here to see what's going on unless I'm needed. Are you needed tonight?" Sara asked Doug.

She had to hand it to both Jessica and Doug. They had kept what looked to be a budding romance secret from their classmates until now. There was no way Doug was down here just to see what was going on.

Doug smiled and replied, "Well, maybe not needed, but hopefully, wanted."

Doug and Jessica smiled at each other, and Sara smiled with them. She had some gossip for Hillary tomorrow.

"Definitely wanted. " Jessica replied to Doug and then turned to Sara. " Now you know our little secret, but we can talk about that later. I'm going to try and get some sleep back in the break room. It's been kinda' quiet tonight. We'll see you in morning, Sara." Jessica and Doug slid back down the hall and toward the break room.

Sara turned back to Quincy in his stall.

"You know this means that I won't get much sleep as long as you're here, right?"

Quincy just stood there looking at Sara as if to say he didn't get much sleep either with this breathing problem, so they would both have valid excuses for being ill and hard to get along with.

"Okay, fella', if it's alright with you, I'm going to go home and get some sleep, but I'll see you in the morning bright and early." Sara paused.

"You know if you'll be a good horse, and the meds start working, I'll be able to take you for walks outside, but that's only if you let us do our work, right?" She asked Quincy.

Sara knew she was in the throes of sleep deprivation, but she could have sworn the horse understood her and was looking forward to going to turn out in a couple of days. He seemed satisfied now, so Sara quickly left the clinic and walked back to her truck.

When she pushed the unlock button on her remote, a black blue head shot up, and Sara feared the worst for her upholstery. As she climbed into the truck, she couldn't feel any wet spots on the seats and the bone had not been chewed into a thousand pieces. It seemed both her patient and her dog had given her a break. Sara settled into the truck as the pup climbed across the console, into the driver's seat, and onto her lap.

"It's going to be a long week, Jake. I hope you're up to the challenge."

As Sara begin stroking his head and put her truck in drive, she muttered, "I hope I'm up to the challenge."

Chapter 16

When Sara and Jake arrived home, she let Jake run around a few minutes outside in case he needed to relieve his bladder. Sara's exhaustion had quickly superseded her anxiety about Quincy soon after she had exited the clinic doors, and the drive home had seemed much longer than the drive to the clinic.

Jake signaled to Sara he had enough of the outdoors and nightlife, so she and the little pup went upstairs. She didn't even bother changing back into her pajamas. She would be up again in less than three hours - there was no need.

Sara lifted Jake in the bed, and set her alarm. Jake had no trouble falling asleep this time, and before Sara could close her eyes, his steady breathing was pushing out soft wisp of air that landed on her ears tickling her insides. Sara turned her head, closed her eyes, and for the second time that night, she slept. This time, she also dreamed.

In her dream, Sara was standing on the bank of a large river. Water dripped from the leaves of the many trees that surrounded Sara on the river's edge, and the grass was soggy underneath her feet. The river roared by her in an angry path downstream. From the swell of the river and the muddy bank around her, Sara knew that the river was close to flooding.

Thunderheads boomed above her and lightning streaked the sky. Gusts of wind surged by, but at this moment in her dream, the rain had stopped.

Sara looked past the river and to the other bank, which seemed miles away. Standing there, in a perfect semi-circle were horses of every age, color, and size. They were all looking at Sara with ears pricked forward at attention. What must have been the leader of the band began to paw at the rain- soaked ground while shaking his head fiercely back and forth. He looked at Sara and began to snort and blow. He reared with his powerful front legs reaching out and pawing at the stormy air.

The others stood quietly allowing their leader to voice a cumulative disgust at the intruder, Sara. They were not afraid of her - they didn't want her at the river. Sara shuddered at their obvious loathing and was relieved that, in her dream, she was on this side of the river and not where the strange band of wild horses stood.

As if to add to Sara's discomfort and unease, a large drop of rain fell from the brimming heavens and splattered squarely on Sara's nose. A thunderclap again sounded, only this time, it shook the earth where Sara stood. She turned to find shelter in the trees from the upcoming downpour, and, as she did, her feet slipped on the soggy ground and surrounding mud.

She felt herself falling, and she couldn't be sure if the roar in her ears was because of the rain that was now pouring down, or the river raging with the storm. Somehow, though, she knew that if she fell in that river, instead of it carrying her downstream, it would carry her to the other bank - the bank where the band of horses stood.

Sara could not break her fall and down into the river she slid. As the water engulfed her, she was able to fight the current that was trying to pull her under and break the surface of the water. She was now halfway to the other side of the river, and the leader stood on the edge of the bank waiting for the river to carry her to him.

The current took Sara down again, and again she was able to swim to the surface. As she forced her head above the water, she looked up just in time to realize that she had made it to the other bank. The leader of the band had risen on his back feet at the water's edge to welcome Sara with a powerful strike of both front hooves squarely to the skull.

Sara set straight up in bed. She was fully awake and in her warm, dry bed, but she still placed her hand on the sleeping Jake to assure herself that she was not on the river's edge. Sara hated these dreams. She used to have them all the time as a child. Dreams with such clarity that when she did wake from them, it would always take her a minute to decide which was real - this world or the one from which she had just come. What made these dreams even worse was that sometimes, they came true.

"You know that dream is not going to come true, so just go back to sleep. There is no way you are going to be standing on a river bank in a storm with a band of wild horses on the other side waiting to stomp you to pieces. Now, go back to sleep."

Sara's little talk with herself had roused Jake. He looked at Sara with one eye open and one eye shut trying to decide if she was talking to him, or to herself. He had been around long enough to know that either was possible.

Sara turned to look at the clock which read four a.m. and then snuggled back under the covers, patted him on his head, and went back to sleep, satisfying Jake that indeed, she had been talking to herself again, and it was time to close the one eye and follow her example.

Chapter 17

The alarm woke them up at six a.m. Sara jumped out of bed and got ready for the day. The shower was heaven after the last couple of days, and when she got out, she felt like a person again. After taking care of Jake and going through her morning routine, Sara returned to the clinic.

Quincy was waiting for her when she arrived at seven. To Sara's surprise, he seemed better. A quick exam indeed confirmed her patient was improved, and even the impartial voice inside her head was impressed - just a little. The voice still swayed on the side of impending doom, but Sara decided not to listen. She made sure Quincy was comfortable, treated her other patients, and then made her way down to the break room to catch up on her patient's records and get ready for the rest of the day.

Jessica and Doug were there slamming down coffee while Hillary was reviewing one of her own patient's record and looking up facts in the textbook she had sprawled across her lap.

"Well, how'd he do last night after I left, Jessica?" Sara asked.

"He did fine, Sara. It was like he just soothed out after he saw you last night. I didn't hear another peep from him. I got to get some sleep last night, and I haven't checked him this morning. He doin' okay?"

"He actually looks better which, I gotta' say, surprises me."

"Why shouldn't he be doing better, Sara?" Hillary piped in, "The great horse doctor to be has put her mind to getting him well. He'll do fine."

"Yeah, right. I wish I were as sure as you are. My instinct tells me we still have a long way to go."

"Then to tell you the truth, I'd be worried, too." Hillary replied while never looking up from the textbook. She didn't have to. She knew exactly what Sara meant.

Hillary had it, too, and Sara knew she did - the instinct. While working in the clinics, Sara could tell which of her classmates had that natural instinct to take care of animals and which ones didn't. Sara often times wondered why her classmates that didn't possess this talent ever ended up in veterinary medicine. She also wondered if they were going to be happy with the profession they had chosen.

No matter what the books, clinical tests, or the specialist told you, and not all of the specialist had the instinct either, it seemed that some possessed a feeling deep in their guts that let them know how that animal really was. The bloodwork could look great, the animal improving and everything looked good, but if you had the instinct, and it said all was not right, you would come back to check that animal long after most had gone home. Most of time, you would find that things had changed and weren't exactly as the tests or textbooks or specialist had said they would be.

The animals in the large and small animal intensive care units were constantly monitored, but just like in human medicine, once an animal got released into the wards and didn't have regular treatments, that animal might only be checked two or three times a day.

Sara's classmates with the "instinct" were easy to recognize. They were the ones she met in the parking lot and in the clinic after hours shyly getting out of their cars or walking the halls to go and check their patients. They might find something as simple as an IV line that had been chewed through to an animal that was on a downward spiral and needed medical attention as soon as possible.

Sometimes the instinct was too cautious - the glass always half empty syndrome. You would come back to a completely happy animal looking at you through a cage door or a stall wondering why you were there. Most of the time, however, the instinct was right on the money.

Sara had some brilliant classmates who did not possess the instinct, and they and their patients had suffered because of it in clinical rotations. With all their book sense, they had missed subtle clues from the animals – clues that turned into problems. She wondered how these classmates would do in practice relying only on science because no matter what anyone told you, veterinary practice was also an art.

Dr. Summers walked in and successfully shattered Sara's reverie of instinct and art and science. With one eye on her patient's chart and the other on the resident, Sara tried to tell from Dr. Summers' body language if today would be a good day or a bad day. She soon got her answer.

"Has everyone checked and treated their patients' this morning?" Julia Summers asked.

"Ummm, we still have about an hour before rounds, don't we, Dr. Summers?" Doug asked.

"So, you should already have your patients treated and records up-to-date this morning. Where is the rest of the rotation? Are they even here yet?" Julia asked.

"We don't know, ma'am, but we better be treating our patients, and we'll look for the others." Hillary lied.

"Okay, y'all get your patients set, find your classmates, and meet me at the Taylor horse's stall by nine sharp. We've got several patients to see this morning, and I can't be waiting for y'all to waste the morning away in the break room drinking coffee. Get going," Dr. Summers ordered.

"Yes, ma'am," they all squeaked in unison, and like herding buffalo, quickly exited the break room.

"Going to be a good day down at the old salt mines today. I can tell already. My patient load is pretty light, though. Anybody need any help?" Doug asked.

"Sure, come with me." Jessica smiled as she took Doug by the hand, and the two of them went off down the corridor to the patients Jessica had received last night on emergency.

"Looks like something's getting started there, doesn't it?" Hillary asked Sara with a sly grin.

"Getting started? It's already begun. He was here last night with her when Quincy was giving everybody a fit."

"He was?"

"Yep, and she pretty much admitted to it. Why else would he be here when he's not on emergency and doesn't have any night treatments? I'd be at home, but he was here."

"Oooh, we better keep an eye on them. I hope it works for them. I like them both. You saw how she took his hand, didn't you?"

"How could you miss it? I think it's been going on awhile. They've just been good about hiding it. We'll have to see how it works out."

"I know we could gossip about this romance thing longer, but did I hear her say you had to come back last night?"

"Quincy wouldn't let Jessica and Doug do his treatment. He was throwing a fit, so she called me."

"Everything go okay once you go here?"

"He calmed down as soon as he heard my voice, and Jess said he did fine the rest of the night."

"Sara, I'm worried about you on this one. Keep your distance. Remember, you have to be objective."

"You're crazy, Hillary. I have no idea what you are talking about."

"Whatever, Sara. Just watch it. I can tell you really like this horse, and you and I both know the odds aren't for him. We are going to lose some, and it's easier if we aren't attached to them. That's all I'm going to say about it. Anyway, I've got to go treat my momma cow that is never glad to see me. You need any help?" Hillary asked.

"I think I got it, but thanks. You need any help with your cow?" Sara replied.

"If you hear me yelling, you know she's got me pinned. If you hear a big thump and no yelling, you know I'm probably unconscious." Hillary laughed as she left Sara and made her way to the food animal corridor of the clinic.

Chapter 18

Sara looked in at Quincy to see him munching on the food she had given him first thing this morning before getting his medications together. He had heard her coming, and as she poked her head around the corner, he whinnied.

"We are feeling better aren't we, fella? If you keep on improving, we might even get to go outside this afternoon. I heard on the radio that it's going to be a nice, spring day. Wouldn't that be awesome?"

Quincy continued to munch as Sara gave him his meds. He gave her no trouble and before she knew it, Dr. Summers and the crew were at the stall.

As they all discussed Quincy, he looked on with mild interest. Even though he was feeling better, everyone was in agreement that follow-up bloodwork and radiographs were needed. Depending on the results of those tests, other tests might be done. Sara would pull the blood and send it to the lab before lunch, and she knew Seth would come get Quincy for his radiographs before lunch while she saw other patients. Hopefully, Quincy would let Seth do his job without tranquilization today. As Dr. Summers, Sara, and the group all decided on the next course of action for Quincy, Dr. Sneed was nowhere to be seen. Sara doubted if he even remembered the horse.

Before going to their next case, Sara had a question for Dr. Summers.

"Dr. Summers, do you think we might be able to get Quincy some turn out time today?"

"That's up to you and his test results, Sara. If you think he's up to it, and you can work it in between your incoming cases and scheduling his test, go for it. We've talked about how allergens and dust exacerbate his condition. Do you think it would be good for him to go outside on a spring day like today?"

Sara had done her research and had been waiting for this question.

"Most horses with COPD do much better if they are outside. The allergen concentration is lower outside, even on a day like today. I not only think it would help his condition, but I think it would help his spirits, too." Sara replied.

"Good answer." Dr. Summers said with a hint of a smile. "Let's go on to our next case. Doug, I believe this one is yours."

So it went for another hour. They all presented their patients, their problems, and they all discussed possible treatment options, why and how those treatments worked, and the expected outcomes. Even though Julia Summers had been in a foul mood earlier this morning, the cases, the questions, and the correctness and efficiency with which the students answered, made her day much brighter.

Julia only had one more week with these students, and they were doing well. This was a good group, and that made things so much easier for Julia. They did their research, they filled out their records, and they took care of their jobs. If Julia were honest with herself, it was the same with most groups. It's just that in the last rotation, none of the students were interested in large animal medicine and were just going through the motions to get through the rotation. In one sense, Julia understood. Small animal practice offered better salaries, more time off, and much better working conditions.

On the other hand, because of her love of horses and veterinary medicine, Julia couldn't understand why some of these students never even considered large or mixed animal practice. There were rewards in this type of work that could not be measured in dollars or vacation time.

Either way, Julia was relieved that she had some students in this rotation that actually wanted to touch a horse or cow when they graduated. It was obvious that Sara's and Hillary's interest and enthusiasm had spread through the whole rotation. Julia wasn't naive enough to believe that any of the other students in the rotation would be interested in large animal practice after graduating, but the dynamics of the whole group in the last three weeks had made teaching them much easier, and when they were so prepared for her questions and all the animals were so well taken care of, Julia knew that, at the very least, she was doing the best she could at her job.

On to a new day and more work to be done, so Julia needed to start assigning cases for the day. She had several animals coming this morning, but she also needed several students to go on farm calls with the ambulatory clinician.

"Doug, you, Jessica, and Josh need to ride with the ambulatory clinician today, and Sara and Hillary need to stay with me. Dr. Rodriquez is on ambulatory and will be waiting for you. There are several farms he has to visit today."

Sara and Hillary smiled at each other. Most of the time, Dr. Summers made sure the young women were split up in their duties. Sara and Hillary figured she didn't want them working together because they were good friends and might not put the client and patient's interest first. Julia had another reason.

She knew the girls would talk about their cases with each other, and in this way, both girls would learn more than if they shared certain duties in the clinic. Julia had no doubt what came first with Sara and Hillary, and as the rotation was nearly over, she found herself having complete confidence in the two students and their abilities.

Either way, Sara and Hillary were thrilled to both be in the clinics today and couldn't wait to see what was on the appointment book.

"You ready?" Sara asked Hillary.

"You know it." Hillary replied.

"Let's go up to the front desk and see what's waiting on us."

Chapter 19

At the front desk, two equine clients were already waiting to be seen. Hillary picked up one chart and Sara the other. They both took a minute to go over the charts and then Hillary directed her client to Exam Room one while Sara asked Mr. McPhee to meet her in Exam Room two.

Sara's new client was Mr. Roddy McPhee, and by just looking at him, she could tell she was in for an amusing and possibly frustrating morning. Roddy was about forty and looked like he had just stepped out of an old Western movie. His spindly legs were bowed in an almost comical arch and clad in skintight Wrangler jeans. His belt buckle must have weighed at least twenty pounds and the glare from all the silver and gold in the buckle made Sara wish for a pair of sunglasses.

Above the jeans, he wore a brown Western shirt that looked like a throw back from some country singer, and on his head, a Stetson cowboy hat. His boots were not worn or rugged nor were his spurs, which jangled every time he took a step. Sara had her doubts about how much of a cowboy this cowboy really was.

"Hello, Mr. McPhee. My name is Sara, and I'll be the student on Buck's case today." She almost giggled as she extended her hand out to Roddy.

"Well, I'll tell you little lady, we ain't gonna be doin' no high priced medicine crap with this horse of mine. I already know the problem, and I figure y'all so advance up here, one test oughtta' let me know if that's what he's got or not."

"Do you mind if I ask you a couple of questions before we do our test, Sir?" Again, it was all Sara could do to stifle a giggle, but she knew she was coming off earnest to Roddy. That clinical demeanor she had been taught came in handy in more ways than one.

"You ain't askin' me no questions, and I don't want nobody touchin' my horse except to pull blood on him for this test, understand?" Roddy had suddenly turned surly and loud, and Sara's amusement at the situation turned to a small burning ember of anger just as fast.

"That's fine, sir. If you won't allow me to touch your horse, I need to go speak with a clinician. You can go ahead and unload him."

"Fine! He'll be right in, and you tell that clinician - only one test."

Sara could feel her eyes narrowing and almost tell the vein that ran down the middle of her forehead was becoming visible. No matter how much she masked her emotion, any one that knew her knew that when the vein became visible, she was angry, and people like Roddy made her very angry.

Sara had met many cowboys through her life and as far as she could tell, it was just like in the Westerns. There were good cowboys and there were bad cowboys and there weren't many in between. Sara's father was a good cowboy. He was a good man who loved horses. He didn't have to wear sparkly clothes or tight jeans to make him feel like he could handle a horse or make a statement about his ability. An old ragged cowboy hat and a good pair of boots were all he needed.

The "bad" cowboys usually always wore clothes that pronounced to the world that they rode or worked with horses whether they really did or not. Most were loud, obnoxious, little boys who were trying to be men and the opportunity to be able to dominate a thousand pound animal just stroked their testosterone filled egos.

They usually didn't care about family and thought of women in much the same way they thought about their animals. The world was there to serve them – woman or beast. They were usually selfish, immature, and had low self-esteem. Why else would they be so loud and boisterous about their make- believe accomplishments. If they talked loud enough and long enough, maybe someone, anyone, would believe they were somebody.

Sara despised this type of man, and she had seen plenty. Coming from a small town and going to a small undergraduate college, Sara had seen her friends get mixed up with these boys who turned into men, and it hadn't been pretty. Most were ignorant, hardheaded fools that listened to no one and did exactly as they pleased. The fact that these men got themselves in all kind of trouble and suffered from their stubbornness didn't bother Sara a bit. What did bother her, though, were the people and the animals that suffered because these men "owned" them.

Sara went to get Dr. Summers and apprise her of the situation. Luckily, Dr. Summers was coming around the corner.

"Dr. Summers, we've got a good one in Exam Room two."

Julia saw the vein in Sara's forehead and knew that her bad day turned better day had just turned bad again.

"Really, Sara, go ahead."

"Well, Cowboy Joe in there says he's pretty sure he knows what's wrong with his horse, and doesn't want us to touch it except to pull blood and run a test. He has not enlightened me with what tests he wants run, and I bet he doesn't even know. He doesn't want to answer any questions about the horse or for us to do a physical exam. He just wants this one test, whatever it is, and that's all. Plus, he got pretty ill, and he yells."

"Hmmmm," Julia replied, "This is going to be fun."

Julia, in all her five foot nothing glory entered the exam room with her chin and chest jutted out. It looked to Sara as if Julia had grown five inches in five minutes.

"Mr. McPhee, I'm Dr. Summers, and Sara tells me that you have brought your horse for us to pull blood and run one test. Can I ask you what test you want?"

"Well, I don't know for sure, but it's some test you can run on his blood to tell why he's gimping on the front, right leg."

"Mr. McPhee, I'm not aware of one single blood test that can be done to determine a lameness in a horse. Sara also tells me that you don't want us to ask you any questions about his lameness or do a physical exam. Is this correct?"

"That's right, little miss. I want that one test, whatever it is, and that's it. Maybe you should ask one of the real doctors what that test is."

Sara almost felt sorry for Roddy McPhee - almost. He had no idea what a storm he had just summoned on his head.

Julia glared at the man, and Sara could swear Roddy squirmed. The old cowboy might be stupid, but he could sure tell an angry woman when he saw one, and he had made Julia Summers angry.

"Mr. McPhee, I am a real doctor, and as an equine internist, you probably don't understand those words - a veterinarian that specializes in horses, I assure you there is no such test. Why don't I just fill you in on how things work around here, Mr. McPhee. Will that be okay?" Julia spoke in a low, menacing tone. She didn't wait for his response.

"We are a referral veterinary hospital. That basically means that a practicing veterinarian refers the clients and patient to us because they need help with diagnosing or treating the patient. From your records, I see that you don't have a regular veterinarian, and I will go so far as to say you don't have a regular veterinarian because no veterinarian will put up with you. Now, I'll make this very clear, so you can understand. First, Mr. McPhee, our students here are the next generation of veterinarians, and you treat them with respect because if you do decide that we will diagnose and treat your horse, it will be our students who will take care of your animal, and as their resident, I will not tolerate any disrespect towards my students.

Second, we will work with you any way we can, but we are not a fast food restaurant where you order your tests from a menu. We are a veterinary hospital, and we are here to do what is best for the animal while also helping the client. If you will not answer our questions about your horse, let us touch your horse, examine your horse, and run whatever tests we need to run on your horse to find out what may be the problem with your horse, then we don't need you as a client.

I am sure you think you know what's wrong with this horse, and I'm also sure you have quite a bit of experience with horses, but may I be so bold as to offer the possibility that there is a chance, especially since this so-called blood test does not exist, that you are wrong, and that we, as veterinarians, who specialize in horses and see many horses with problems every day, every week, and every year, might know just a smidgin' bit more than you do about a horse?"

Sara didn't know how Julia said all that without taking a breath, but she did. It was great. It was all Sara could do not to laugh out loud as she watched Roddy McPhee sink further and further into the corner of the room. Sara's anger had vanished and her respect for Dr. Summers had risen to a new level as she watched this spunky woman stand up to this man.

"Now, having said all that, Mr. McPhee, I only have one question for you. Do you want us to look at your horse or not?" Julia asked.

Roddy stood there looking like a whipped dog for a second, and then Sara saw it in his eyes and his face. Dr. Summers had startled him at first with her anger and her honesty. He knew every word she said was true, and for a minute, Sara thought they might just see this ole' cowboy do the right thing but then that look of stupidity and defiance begin to show in his eyes. Sara could almost read his mind, and she knew exactly what he was thinking.

Who the hell did they think they were talking to someone as important as him like this? These were a bunch of women, and everybody knows women don't know nothin' about no horse - not really. What kind of place is this where you come in and just because you talk a little rough to the help, you get an earful like this? Buck needed some medical attention, so Roddy could make some money, but it wasn't worth all this. He'd find somebody that would do what he wanted, and it would probably be a lot cheaper than these yahoos. Bunch of crazy women. Then, Roddy spoke.

"No, ma'am, you ain't lookin' at my horse. He don't need none of your big shot medicine anyway. I'll just run him hurt and don't care. If he gets hurt worse where I can't use him, I'll just shoot him myself. Ya'll ain't talking to me that way. I know what's best for my horse whether I'm a veterinarian or not, so I'm just going to load this old boy up and see if I can't find someone else to look at him."

"Good, Mr. McPhee. We hope you find someone that will oblige you." Dr. Summers retorted, turned on her heel, and exited the room, and Sara followed.

"Go up to the reception area and tell the front desk to not charge Mr. McPhee. I imagine he'll just load his horse up and haul it out of here anyway, but just in case he doesn't, I don't want a scene up there either." Julia directed Sara.

"Yes, ma'am. Whew, you sure told him." Sara said with a slight grin that quickly faded as Julia turned to face her.

"Yes, I did, Sara, which sometimes is not the best thing to do, but no one, and I mean no one is going to order my students around but me, and no one is going to demand that I perform a service as a veterinarian just because that's what they want done. There are many Mr. McPhee's out there, and you will soon have your chance to meet them. Just remember that not everyone has the same advantage of picking and choosing their cases as we do here at the university. In the near future, you will probably have to deal with a Roddy McPhee, and you may need to handle it differently than I did. Understand?"

"Frankly, no, I don't understand. I think you handled that beautifully, and I hope I have the guts to handle it the same way when I'm in practice."

"Well, Sara, that will probably depend on who you work for and where you work. Most young practices and veterinarians can't afford to turn clients away, but as you practice longer, you will see that some clients aren't worth the heartache and the worry. The philosophy of the practice owner, whether you want to work there or not, and what kind of medicine you want to practice will all determine if you turn the Roddy McPhees of this world away or not, and if you don't turn them away, I didn't give you the best example in there of how to deal with them."

"Don't worry about that, Dr. Summers. Like you said, I'll have plenty of time to figure out how I'm going to deal with the Roddy McPhees of this world later, but right now, I'm going to run up to the front desk to let them know and start another case. Thanks for the advice, and thanks for taking up for us."

"No problem, Sara, just call me when you need me." And with that, Julia Summers disappeared down the hall.

Chapter 20

Sara's next client was waiting in the reception area. From the chart, Sara saw he was a dairy farmer who had brought one of his milking cows. Mr. Young was a man who Sara guessed to be in his thirties. He was about six feet tall with wide shoulders and the beginnings of a pooch at his mid-riff. His dairy was in the Knoxville area, so he had not had to travel far, but Sara smiled to herself as she noticed him dozing in his chair. It was only 10:30, but from Sara's estimate, Mr. Young probably milked at 4am and 4pm. That would mean he probably rose about 3am every morning. Sara would have been dozing, too.

"Mr. Young, Sir?" Sara called.

Mr. Young's head snapped up, and he woke with a little start. "Yes, ma'am?"

"I'm Sara, and if you want to go ahead and pull around back, I'll help you unload your cow."

"Okay, Sara, I'll be around in a minute."

As Sara walked back to the food animal ward, she didn't think she would have any trouble from Mr. Young. Maybe it was in the way he ambled to the doors to unload or the way his checked shirt tail had worked its way out the back of his jeans making him look like a big kid, but whatever it was, Sara felt that Mr. Young would do what was needed to get his cow well. Not only would he do whatever was needed, but Sara also felt he would be a perfect gentleman through it all, as most dairymen were.

Sara had no prior experience with dairies before she had come to vet school. In West Tennessee, dairies were not as common as beef cattle operations. The more she learned about the dairy industry and how hard these farmers worked, the more she respected them. The big corporate dairies that were taking over did not quite have the same effect on Sara, but the smaller farmers repeatedly won Sara's respect.

Who in their right mind would get up at 3am every morning, go out into the cold or heat in the dark, get up cows, and milk one hundred head of cattle? After milking, there were chores on the farm, feeding calves, treating sick cows, checking dry cows, and the list went on and on, and no matter if you were done or not, the cows got milked at least once more and possibly twice more that same day, and then you got to get up the next day and do it all over again - weekend, holiday or not.

Most dairymen Sara knew took very few vacations and worked like dogs. It didn't matter if you were sick, hurt, or just plain worn down; the cows had to be milked. Either you milked them, or you had to hire someone else or a couple of some ones to milk them. And for all your backbreaking work, dairymen hardly ever got any thanks. After all, the grocery store makes milk, right?

Lost in her thoughts, Sara had walked to the unloading door before she knew it. Mr. Young was putting a halter on the cow.

"Mr. Young, if you want to wait a minute, I'll set up the cattle chute and we can run her in the head gate."

"Oh, you won't need the chute and head gate, Sara. Ole' Bessie is halter broke, and she'll stand tied just fine. I'll just tie her to that gate there, and you can examine her."

"Okay, Mr. Young, whatever you say." Sara replied.

Mr. Young got Bessie tied, and Sara began asking him questions about her history and the nature of her illness. She asked things like when did she calve, was she still eating, how much milk was she giving, did she seem to be chewing her cud, etc. The more questions she asked, the bigger the smile on Mr. Young's face got.

"You reckon you already know what's wrong with my cow, Sara?" Mr. Young asked.

"From the grin on your face, I reckon you know what's wrong with your cow, too, Mr. Young."

"Well, now, Sara, don't you figure you need to do a physical exam?"

"Sure, Mr. Young, that'll let us know for sure."

"If I was you, Sara, I'd try listening to her left side and thumpin' it a bit. You might get lucky and hear something like when you thump a real full basketball."

Sara performed her physical exam, and sure enough she heard that signature ping on the cow's left side.

"Well, Mr. Young, I'll go get a resident now since we've both figured out your cow has a LDA." Sara said with a smile.

"I think that would be a good idea, Sara. I'll be right here with Bessie." Mr. Young replied.

An LDA was short for left displaced abomasum or in common terms, a stomach that had moved where it didn't need to be, and Bessie showed all the classic signs on physical exam. It was a relatively common problem with dairy cattle that did, however, require surgery, so as soon as Dr. Summers had confirmed the diagnosis, Bessie would be moved to the surgery rotation.

Mr. Young had known Bessie would probably need surgery. Sara had seen he was a long time client on his chart. Even though he knew Bessie should have been seen by surgery, he had still let Sara ask all those questions, do her physical exam, and had even given her a hint on the cow's problem.

Why? Because he was a patient man, and he had manners, and he knew the students who were here today would be the veterinarians that were practicing tomorrow. He wanted to make sure he helped them any way he could. His way to help was to bring his cows, not act like he knew everything, but to patiently wait and watch.

Sara went to the phone and paged Dr. Summers who appeared in about two minutes.

"Okay, Sara, what do we have?"

"Pretty sure it's a LDA, Dr. Summers. The cow belongs to a Mr. Young. He's from around here and has been here several times."

"Oh, it's Brian's cow?" Julia asked.

"I didn't look at the first name, ma'am."

Dr. Summers thumbed through the chart.

"Yeah, it's Brian's cow. Did he tell you what was wrong with her before you had a chance to figure it out?"

"No, ma'am, he just gave me a hint, but I think I already had it figured out."

"Well, let's go see him."

Julia approached Brian with a wide smile and an outstretched hand.

"It's good to see you, Brian."

"Good to see you, too, Julia, but I think they should have put me in the surgery rotation instead of medicine."

"You're right. Why didn't you say anything up front? You knew what was wrong with your cow."

"Well, Julia, that's not entirely true. I thought I knew what my cow had, and this young lady has assured me that I am right, but I know how things work around here, and I wasn't going to put up no fuss. Whoever wants to listen to ole' Bessie is fine with me. I know y'all fix her even if it might take a little while."

"Okay then Brian, just let me do a quick exam, and I'll get someone from surgery down here."

"Go right ahead, Julia, but I think this young lady has it pretty well pinned down."

"I'm sure she does, Brian, but you know the protocol."

So Mr. Young and Sara stood back and let Dr. Summers do her physical exam. Mr. Young was quietly leaning against the gate with his fingers scratching the top of Bessie's head, and Bessie didn't mind at all.

Even though Bessie was not a pet, one could see Mr. Young was concerned about Bessie's welfare. Sara knew that if Bessie was a good milker, the cow made money for Mr. Young, and high-milking dairy cows were an expensive commodity. Besides the monetary value of the cow, though, Sara also knew that Mr. Young had a kind heart and hated to see any animal hurt or sick.

Maybe it was the way he leaned against the fence or the way he had slyly given Sara her "hint', but whatever it was; Sara knew this man standing before her was of a completely different caliber than her first client of the day. Mr. Young had kind eyes and when he smiled, it was a sheepish grin.

He was slow and steady in his movements, and Sara felt he was also slow to anger and had an easy, steady temperament. This man was a hard worker, an honest man, and a man that, with his chosen profession, probably had a hard time in life, but Sara bet he never complained.

Unlike Roddy McPhee who was an arrogant fool without a clue, Mrs. Young had known what was wrong with his cow, but never once, had he overstepped his bounds. He was respectful and thoughtful about everything he said or did. Sara wished she saw a thousand Mr. Youngs a day, and if she were honest with herself, she would admit there were a lot more Mr. Youngs out there than Roddy McPhees. Just like everything else, however, you always remember the bad more than you remember the good.

"Brian, Sara, you were both right. Sara, let's get a student from the surgery rotation to have a look at Bessie, and Brian, we'll have your cow fixed up pretty soon." Julia said as she finished her exam.

"Thanks, Julia, I appreciate it, and Sara?"

"Yes, sir?"

"Good job. Hope you're plannin' on doing mixed animal or large animal practice when you get done here in May. Us farmers could use more vets out there."

"Mr. Young, that's exactly what I plan to do."

"Good, Sara. Maybe I'll see you next time, and Julia, it was good to see you again."

"You, too, Brian. Take care of yourself and your cows." Julia replied.

"I will, Julia."

Sara and Julia left the food animal ward. It took Sara about five minutes to find Will, one of her classmates on the large animal surgery rotation. Dr. Summers had gone to lunch and instructed Sara to do so when she finished with Brian and Bessie.

"Hey, Will, I got a patient for you." Sara called out to Will.

"Gosh, Sara, I was just going to lunch, and I'm starving. Why do you medicine people always do this to me?" Will whined.

"Get over it, Will. It's a good one. You'll enjoy it. The cow has a LDA."

"Well, why didn't you say that in the first place, Sara? I haven't even come close to seeing one of those yet. This'll be pretty cool. I've just got to find Dr. Gibson and get him to look at it, too. You already switched it up front at reception?"

"I've got to get some blood from one of my patients and take it to the lab. I'll tell reception on my up."

"Okay, Sara. Thanks. I'll let you know how it turned out."

Chapter 21

Sara waved as she walked down the hall. She really didn't have a doubt about how it would turn out. An LDA was usually a simple operation, but they didn't get to see many of them because most dairy practitioners would have a veterinarian perform the operation in the field. It wasn't considered a referral case. So, unless a student was with one of the ambulatory clinicians that did the day-to-day farm work and got to see one, most students went through all of clinics without seeing this procedure.

When they got out into practice and into a case like this, the student would have to call the experienced veterinarians they worked with to help them on one or two before they could go on their own. Once she got into practice, Sara was sure there would be a lot of things that would be that way, and she just hoped she ended up with an understanding and patient boss.

The interns, residents, and clinicians assured all of the students that most veterinary practitioners would help them through their first couple of years of practice. It benefitted the student because they didn't feel as if they were being thrown out to fend for themselves, and it benefitted the practitioner to ward off malpractice suits and legal fees.

Sara wondered how many people really thought that when you got that degree, you were ready and able to do everything that veterinary practice required, because she knew she wouldn't be, especially as a mixed animal practitioner. There were simple things she had not seen or been a part of since being in vet school because most of the time, just like Quincy, they were sent cases that practicing veterinarians had already given their best shot. Brian and his cow were the exception.

Sara was just glad she had worked at the animal clinic at home during her summers between her first and second years in vet school. She had learned an enormous amount since she had walked through the doors of the veterinary college four years ago, but she had also learned an enormous amount in the day-to-day practice at the veterinary clinic at home.

Sara had not grown up around cattle, but they saw plenty at the practice at home. She may have learned every anatomical part of the cow, the physiology of the cow, diseases of the cow, and everything else about a cow from the professors in vet school, but Sara had learned how to handle a cow, how to herd a cow, and how to avoid getting squished by a cow from the veterinary technician at home who had worked at auction barns and feedlots since he was fourteen years old.

Sara had also seen clients like Roddy McPhee at home and Brian, but there weren't many clients like Judy where Sara lived. Most of the people at home didn't make that kind of money or have horses like Quincy. Most of the people at home were people just like her parents. They were lucky if they made it through high school and were now working in factory jobs to support their families. They didn't have a lot of options.

Besides working at the clinic at home during the summers during vet school, Sara had also been able to work at the one big factory at home through her summers during college. Working in temperatures over 100 degrees, shift work, and the resigned faces of many of the people that worked there, cemented Sara's ambition to become a veterinarian and probably had a lot to do with her work ethic and tenacity in the clinics. She had always known what she wanted to be, and come hell or high water, she was going to be a veterinarian.

Sara smiled as she realized that in two short months, her dream would come true. The closer she got to graduation, the more and more she thought about home. She had talked with the veterinarians at home about coming back to practice there. They didn't think the clinic could support three veterinarians, but one day, they felt it would, and when that day came, they had promised Sara she had a job.

Sara had been able to find her first job about an hour away from home. The veterinarian there seemed very nice, and she would be much closer to her family than she was now. One day, however, she knew she would return home and practice veterinary medicine.

Chapter 22

Sara started toward Quincy's stall and saw Stephanie with blood tubes in her hand.

"I got your blood from Quincy, Sara. I didn't know how long you would be with Mr. Young, and I knew it needed to go to the lab. I'm headed that way." Stephanie said.

"Thanks, Stephanie. I'm headed to lunch, so I don't mind taking it if you have something else you need to do." Sara offered.

"Actually, that would work great for me. There are a couple more things I could get done down here if you could run it up." Stephanie handed the blood to Sara. "Hope you get some good results from your horse. He looks quite a bit better."

"He does, doesn't he?" Sara was pleased. "Do you know if they've taken the x-rays yet today?"

"Yeah, they came and got him right after rounds, and he did fine. I think Seth had to give him a little something to calm him down, but not much. He's wide awake right now." Stephanie informed Sara.

"I'm not going to the stall then. I've got to treat him at two anyway, and sometimes when he sees me, it's hard to get away from him."

"I'd get some lunch while the getting was good if I was you, Sara."

"I think you're right. Thanks again."

"Sure."

Sara made her way upstairs, dropped off the blood, and was walking to the cafeteria when Seth came up behind her.

"You going to lunch, Sara?" Seth asked.

"Yep. You?"

"On my way," Seth replied.

"Good. You can eat with me and tell me how Quincy's lungs look today. How's radiology anyway?"

"Radiology's fine, Sara, we haven't been very busy today. As for Quincy, there isn't much change from yesterday on his radiographs even though he did act a little better for me than he did yesterday."

"He's better, Seth." Sara said with satisfaction in her voice.

"His lungs still look like crap, Sara."

"Well, lungs of crap or not, he's doing better today. I think we saw him at his worst after that long trailer ride. Once we got him settled and got him on fluids, antibiotics, and started his breathing treatments, he's actually gotten a little spunky. Don't get me wrong, he's not looking to run the Kentucky Derby, but I do think he's probably well enough to have some turn out time this afternoon."

"That's great, Sara, but I'm tellin' you, don't get your hopes up too much on this one. He's a sick boy."

"Seth, I know he feels better today. He's improved a lot from yesterday. A couple of more days with that kind of improvement, and he'll be ready to go home."

"Sara, what did the voice say?"

Sara had been busy getting her standard lunch of a diet coke and peanut butter and crackers, but this question made her pause and look up at him. Seth was a big man, but as Sara turned her disconcerting gaze upon him, he seemed to shrink to a boy. He was looking down at his boots with his eyelids half closed while his fingers were twiddling with the loose string hanging from the pocket of his coveralls.

"Seth, we agreed we wouldn't talk about the voice, didn't we?"

"Yeah, but I'm asking anyway, Sara." Seth continued to twiddle with the string and not look Sara in the eye.

"The voice says there's not much of a chance, Seth. Is that what you wanted to hear?" Sara shot back.

"No, Sara, I just don't want you to get your hopes up. I remember what happened yesterday, how the horse wouldn't let you leave his sight, and Jessica told me what happened last night. You just need to keep your distance on this one, Sara. Listen to your voice. I'm not saying he won't get well, I'm just saying if you get too attached to this horse, you're probably going to regret it. That's all I'm saying. Besides, me and you both know you can't be having an emotional breakdown at the end of clinics." Seth said this last part with a smile and to break the tension.

Sara snorted a laugh and rolled her eyes as she playfully punched Seth on the shoulder. They both knew Sara would not be having an emotional breakdown anytime soon. Seth thought Sara was made of steel, and Sara didn't figure she'd tell him any different. Throughout their classroom and clinical years, it was well known that Sara had never shed a tear.

She just wasn't the crying type. They had all seen plenty of their classmates shed tears whether from stress, bad test scores, patients dying, or various other things, but not once, had anyone ever seen Sara tear up. Sara knew she had to be tough to do what she was going to do, and even if she wasn't as tough as everyone thought, Sara didn't think that was anybody's business but hers.

"Seth, let's talk about something else. I've got to call Mrs. Taylor after lunch and let her know how Quincy's doing. I'd like to forget about all this for fifteen or twenty minutes and just relax. Okay?"

"Sure, Sara, what do you want to talk about?"

"I don't care, just anything except my horse or emotional breakdowns."

"Your horse, huh? Naw, Sara, you're not getting attached at all."

"Shut up, Seth, and change the subject."

"Okay, I'll change the subject. Speaking of Jessica, are her and Doug gettin' it on because it seems their relationship has definitely been evolving over the last several weeks?"

"That's funny because that is exactly what me and Hillary were talking about earlier today. I believe the answer to your question is yes. He was with her last night while she was on emergency. I'm going to have to like someone pretty good to be down here at two in the morning."

"No, kiddin. I stayed with Shelby a couple of times last year, but most of the time, I was snoozin' when she was on emergency."

"How is Shelby, by the way? You two still good?"

"Yep, we're still good. She likes the clinic she's working at, and we try to make time for each other. One thing about it, she knows exactly how this year is for me, so she understands I don't have a lot of time."

"Well, good. I'm glad the clinic monster hasn't got y'all two at odds. It's kinda' funny how this year gets some people together while others, it tears apart, isn't it?"

"Yep, as long as my relationship isn't the one it tears apart."

"I don't think you have anything to worry about, Seth. Shelby's crazy about you."

"Yeah, I know, how can she help herself?" Seth replied with an evil grin. "She knows I'm crazy about her, too. She's my dream come true. Well, enough about me, Sara. I've got to get back to radiology. Dusty is probably wondering where I am. I imagine he's gettin' a little hungry himself."

"Okay, Seth, have a good one."

"You, too, Sara. I'll see you later."

Chapter 23

Sara sat by herself munching on her peanut butter and crackers, and thought about her and Seth's conversation. She had seen many of her classmates old relationships fall apart and new relationships begin. She remembered the guy at the beginning of second year standing in front of the class telling them that he was going to have to leave vet school. He had explained to his classmates that it was either his career or his marriage, and he was going with his marriage.

Sara couldn't remember his name, but she vividly remembered him standing on those steps in the auditorium classroom announcing to his classmates he was leaving and the anguished look on his face. Sara wondered if he had indeed saved his marriage. They would never know.

Seth and Shelby seemed to be doing okay. Shelby had been Seth's vet school big sister. At the end of the first year in vet school, everyone sits down and picks an incoming student to be their little sister or brother. The purpose was to mentor the entering student, let them see old tests, and basically, just get them through the first year.

Shelby had picked Seth and when he had come to Knoxville that August, they had hit it off immediately. They were inseparable until last year when Shelby was going through her clinical year, and Seth was in his third year. Shelby had found little time for Seth that year, but Seth understood. He knew it would be the same for him in his clinical year. Many men wouldn't have understood. Many women didn't understand either.

Sara had come to the conclusion that most relationships that started in vet school whether it was another classmate; someone from another class, or even someone outside the vet school family seemed to work. The relationships that started before one entered vet school were the ones that struggled. Sara had two classmates now that had married before entering vet school, and both of those marriages were seeing hard times.

Sara had talked to one of her classmates about the trouble he was having with his marriage late one night when they were both on emergency. She was on for large animal medicine and he was on the large animal surgery rotation. Levi was a good guy. He never seemed worried and always had a smile on his face. Levi had seemed worried that night, and the smile was gone. Sara could tell something was wrong.

As they had stood out on the loading dock behind the clinic to take a break and let the cold night air refresh their senses, Sara and Levi had begun talking about their cases. Then, they started talking about all the time they had to spend with their cases. Finally, they had talked about all the time they were away from home, and that's when Levi had told Sara about the fight he and his wife had that night.

Levi's wife had accused him of an affair. She couldn't understand why he was always at school unless it was another woman. Levi had been angry at first. After all, he was doing this for both of them, for a better life, for the children they would have one day. She hadn't believed him.

No matter what he said or how hard he tried to explain, she could not imagine the time clinics involved and was sure it was another woman. Listening to his wife that night, Levi told Sara that he knew there was no way she was going to believe him. His anger had turned to frustration and now, his frustration had turned to despair which was evident in his voice and actions that night on the dock.

Levi had spent countless hours, hundreds of thousands of dollars, and four years to get his doctorate in veterinary medicine, and they were all so close. He couldn't turn back now. He was sure when he got home, his wife would be gone, but when they had called with an emergency, he had left anyway. He had no choice.

Sara had tried to comfort him by assuring him that his wife would be there in the morning. She had even offered to talk with his wife, but since his wife thought he was having an affair, they both agreed that wouldn't be the best idea. Sara had no idea how to help Levi, and she knew there was no way she could. Levi's marriage could be one of the many vet school relationship casualties.

Sara had seen him a couple of days later and asked if everything was okay. She could tell from his face that it wasn't even before he filled her in. His wife had indeed been gone that next morning. She had moved four hours away to stay with her mother until they got everything straightened out.

Sara tried to tell him it would be okay, he tried to agree, but they both knew it might not. One of her other classmates, Jane, had gone through the exact same thing less than two months ago. It was just the husband, not the wife moving away.

The problem, as Sara saw it, was simple. Those couples had lives together four years ago. They had done things with each other, spent time together, and had seen each other, at the very least, a couple of hours a day. That had come to a screeching halt when their partner started vet school, and for many, they did not understand - at all.

Sara thought about her classmates that had started relationships in vet school. Those significant others knew, from the very beginning what came first - vet school. If they didn't like it, well they didn't last long. Most of them didn't feel as if they had time for a relationship anyway, but if they found an understanding partner, there was a chance it could work.

If one was fortunate, they would feel the spark with someone who was already in vet school and no explanation was needed. Like Seth and Shelby, both knew the nature of the relationship. Vet school came first, but you had the same goals, the same dreams, and the same ambitions. You understood each other and knew the time and energy it took and all the stress involved. It was the best of both worlds.

Sara had not found that understanding partner in the outside world and the majority of her male classmates were either already in a relationship or she just saw them as friends. Sara had dated some men while in vet school, but as soon as a guy started demanding more time or becoming possessive, she dropped him.

She would have plenty of time for men later, but now she only had time for her career which brought her back to two of the most important males in her life right now - Jake and Quincy. She needed to call Mrs. Taylor before her lunch break was over.

Chapter 24

"Mrs. Taylor?" Sara asked as she held the receiver close to block out the noise from the large animal clinic.

"Sara, is that you? How's Quincy?"

"He's doing better, Mrs. Taylor. After I see some of my patients and get through afternoon rounds, I'm going to take him outside for awhile and let him have some sun and fresh air."

"He's that much better, Sara?"

"Yes, ma'am, he sure is. I think he'll really enjoy being out this afternoon. I think it'll do him good."

"That's wonderful news. I've been worried to death. I knew you would have called if he was worse, but it's just hard waiting by the phone and not knowing what's going on."

"I can sure understand that, Mrs. Taylor, but everything is fine here. If you want me to, I'll call you again this afternoon after Quincy's been outside to let you know how he did."

"That would be great, Sara. I'd love to hear from you again this afternoon, and it sure would help ease my mind."

"No problem. I'm not sure what time it'll be when I'll call, but it'll probably be around five or six. Is that okay with you?"

"I'll be here, and, Sara?"

"Yes, ma'am?"

"Thanks for taking care of my boy."

"You're welcome, ma'am. It's my pleasure."

"I'll be looking forward to hearing from you this evening."

"Okay, ma'am, talk to you then."

Sara hung up the phone and went to check her other patients. They didn't have any other appointments scheduled till late afternoon. She should be able to check them and get Quincy's two o'clock treatment in before she had to see anyone else.

Most of Sara's patients had been discharged yesterday, and she had not admitted any today, so there were only two remaining patients to check. One was a goat that had been very close to death when he had arrived. Parasites had been his problem. Her other patient was a pony who had foundered. Both were doing much better, and Sara was going to recommend they go home tomorrow. Neither required treatment more than once a day since they had been doing so well.

The goat was hilarious, and Sara loved to watch him. When Thumper had first come in, he had no strength and could barely get around. The parasites had robbed him of blood and nutrients. He had been anything but inquisitive, but as they began treating Thumper and he began to improve, his true personality started shining through.

Although many people raised goats to sell, milk, or eat, Thumper was a pet, and it was obvious. He was the ward comedian always into something or running up to you bleating as soon as he saw anyone who might pay him some attention. Today, he saw Sara coming and had somehow managed to get his head stuck in between the rails of his stall door.

"Hello, Thumper, are you going to be able to get out of that yourself, or am I going to have to saw your head off?" Sara questioned the goat with a laugh. "Don't worry. I'll get you out of there."

Sara repositioned Thumper's head, and it easily slid through the railing. She then gave him a quick pat, checked to make sure his water buckets were full and that he had indeed eaten all of his morning feeding.

"I think I'm going to draw a little blood on you to see how you're doing, Thumper. If everything looks good with that, I imagine I'll be sending you home. I've got to go get some help to hold you, though, because I don't think you are going to just stand there for this. I'll be back in a minute."

Sara grabbed some blood tubes and syringes from the workstation and began looking for either a classmate or technician to help with Thumper. She didn't have to look long. Sara spotted Leanne down the hall. She needed to thank Leanne for taking Jake out yesterday anyway, and while she was at it, she'd just ask another favor.

"Hey, Leanne, what're you doing?"

"Come here, Sara, I need a little help." Leanne called back.

Leanne was working on a llama that wasn't happy about being treated at all. Sara stepped inside the stall, took the lead rope that was attached to the halter from Leanne's hand and tried to keep the animal as still as possible while Leanne drew blood from her patient.

"I'm glad you gave me a yell. Lucy here doesn't appreciate this daily ritual of bloodletting, and she's beginning to get a little ornery about it. She knows exactly what I want from her every day, and she's beginning to resent it. If she doesn't go home soon, I'll probably need three or four people to help every time we draw blood."

"Speaking of help, Leanne, my friend, thanks for letting Jake out yesterday. I really appreciate it." Sara said.

"No problem." Leanne replied.

"Did you get to see the LDA I sent to Will at lunch? How'd that go?" Sara asked.

"Yep, got to see it, and it was pretty cool. It went fine." Leanne replied. "By the way, Sara, I need help with something else, too."

"Okay, what is it?" Asked Sara.

"I go on small animal anesthesia next week, so I'll have ICU shifts. You know you will probably have to help me out with Bubbles." Leanne smiled knowingly at Sara.

"Bubbles don't like me, Leanne."

"Bubbles doesn't like anyone, Sara, but she will tolerate you."

Bubbles only tolerated Sara because she didn't have a choice. If she wanted out when her owner was busy, she had to let Sara walk her. Bubbles was an old Boston Terrier that loved no one but Leanne and Leanne loved the old dog with all her heart. Leanne had rescued Bubbles from an animal shelter when Leanne was just a girl and Bubbles was just a puppy. Now, fourteen years later, Leanne had grown into a woman and Bubbles had grown into a grumpy old dog, but the two loved each other completely.

Sara visited Leanne in Building B of the apartment complex quite often last summer when they had first begun their rotations. Leanne's building was right by the pool. The girls had started on the same rotation, so if they had some time off, the pool was where the girls would go. They would spend time by the pool, relax, and end up at Leanne's apartment talking about everything from clinics, to men, to pets, to families.

Sara and Leanne relied on each other heavily when it came to taking care of each other's pets and of each other, but because of their differing schedules as the clinical year had progressed, there were no more days at the pool and not a lot of time talking, but that was okay. Both girls understood.

"Okay, Leanne, I've helped you with this llama, and you know I'll walk mean ole' Bubbles, but you've got to do me a favor." Sara said in a matter of fact manner.

"Sara, I've done you favors." Leanne said dryly.

"I need another." Sara smiled at her friend.

"What?" Leanne was blunt, but that was one of the things Sara loved about her.

"Blood on the goat." Sara was pretty blunt herself.

"Gosh, Sara, you know I don't especially like goats." Leanne whined.

"Hating it for you." Sara replied with a smirk.

"Okay, where and when?"

"Right now and just down the hall. Come on."

"Crap." Leanne followed Sara to Thumper's stall.

Thumper realized he again had an audience and was trying to get his water bucket off the hook, so he could roll it around the stall.

"Okay, I don't like goats in general, but this goat is hilarious. Sometimes when Lucy gives me trouble, I just come down here and watch him to get a laugh." Leanne noted.

"Let's see how hilarious he is when I stick this needle in his neck." Sara replied.

Thumper gave the girls some resistance, but the job was done in no time. Leanne volunteered to take Thumper's blood to the lab since she had to take Lucy's anyway. Sara thanked her again for taking care of Jake and reminded her to call when she needed Sara to take care of Bubbles. Leanne assured her she would.

Sara checked her watch. She had spent too much time talking with Leanne. It was nearly two o'clock and she still had to check her other patient before treating Quincy. Sara hurried down to Dino, the foundered pony's stall. He was munching hay and looked comfortable.

Nothing needed to be done here, and Sara was hoping that once Dino and Thumper were discharged, Quincy would be her only patient in the hospital for the rest of the week. That way, she could concentrate solely on him and hopefully get him ready to go before she left the rotation.

Quincy was waiting for Sara when she arrived with his big head sticking out the stall door. He let out a small whinny when he saw Sara, and Sara let out a satisfied sigh of relief when she saw him. He looked even better than when she had treated him this morning. She got all his medications together and opened the stall door.

"So, are you thinking you may want to go outside this afternoon, Big Boy?"

Quincy stared at Sara with a questioning look as she entered the stall and took a small step back to give Sara some room.

"Don't worry, you'll do fine outside this afternoon. I won't let you do too much, and we'll just take it slow and easy." Sara continued, "Now, just hold still and let me get this stuff in your IV, you'll have to take a puff, and then I'll let you rest. That way, you'll be ready for this afternoon."

As Sara stepped to Quincy's side to treat him, he placed his head on her shoulder. She knew that meant that he trusted her and whatever she asked him to do, he would try. He only moved his head when she asked him to take his breathing treatments. Quincy was by far one of the easiest horses Sara had ever treated, and she knew it wasn't just because he was sick. He was just a one of a kind horse, and Sara knew it. A small knot was forming in the pit of her stomach.

The way Sara saw it; Quincy had complete faith that Sara and the others at the hospital could make him feel better. He knew he already felt much better than yesterday, and he was smart enough, and gentle enough that Sara believed he had figured out what they were doing was indeed helping.

The knot in the pit of her stomach came from worry. Sara had seen how sometimes animals get better, then worse again, then die. Her clinical voice still told her Quincy could do just that, but it also told her that he was much better. Still, she worried.

She finished treating Quincy with the knot still well in place. She stroked his neck and under his chin a couple of times before she stepped out of the stall, and then closed the door. The big head popped out to watch her.

"Don't worry, Buddy, I'll be back in awhile. I'm looking forward to our afternoon out." Sara left Quincy and walked down to look over the charts for the patients that would be coming the rest of the afternoon.

Everything looked pretty straightforward, and Sara didn't foresee any problems. Sara knew Dr. Summers would be checking on them throughout the afternoon, double checking their work and helping them, if needed. It was getting close to her next appointment, so she had better get out there and see if they had arrived.

Chapter 25

The rest of the afternoon Sara saw a cow with pneumonia, a goat with foot rot, and a couple of horses with minor problems. As she had expected, everything went fine. There were no problems from the clients and the patients were diagnosed, treated, and sent home with very little testing or fuss. By the time she had finished with everything, it was just about time for afternoon rounds.

She checked the computer in the break room for Quincy's lab results, and as she had thought, his blood work was better. Even though the x-rays were the same today, the parameters on his blood work had indeed improved. They would definitely get to go outside this afternoon.

Her other classmates had made it back from the farm calls with the ambulatory service, and they all gathered outside the break room waiting on Dr. Summers. She soon appeared.

There weren't many new cases on the ward and since they had all talked exhaustively about the patients that were there, the rounds went quickly. Everyone agreed with Sara that it was time for Dino and Thumper to go home. Doug's patient had some interesting lab work come back, and they all talked about that for a couple of minutes.

Josh, who was always quiet, presented one of his cases they had seen on ambulatory that afternoon. Jessica and Hillary also fielded several questions, but again, most of the cases had been there for a few days, and the students were well versed in the problems their patients had. The last patient to see in rounds was Quincy.

"Well, Sara, we even have some improvement from this morning. That's wonderful." Dr. Summers exclaimed.

"Yes, ma'am. His breathing has definitely gotten better along with his appetite. The x-rays today were pretty much the same as yesterday, but the blood work shows improvement. We're planning on going outside as soon as we finish here." Sara replied.

"What do you think about no improvement radiographically, Sara?" Julia questioned.

"I think it will take a couple more days for us to see anything there, but from his attitude, appetite, and blood work, I think we're on the right track."

"Do you think we need to run any more diagnostic tests right now?"

"I'd kinda' just like to see how he does as long as he's improving, Dr. Summers."

"Okay, Sara, I agree. We just need to keep a close eye on him which I know you will do." Julia then turned her attention to the rest of her students. "Okay, guys, looks like everything is taken care of for the night. Hillary, you know you are on call tonight, so everyone else, let's get our patients treated if they need it, and if not, you're dismissed until the morning. Have a good night."

Sara was sure that was the quickest afternoon rounds of the rotation. Dr. Summers must be tired, as they all were. Even though afternoon rounds went by like a flash, it wasn't quick enough for Sara. She was ready to take Quincy out. After all the students had gone their own way, she grabbed a lead rope from the hook in the hall and headed back to Quincy's stall.

His head was sticking out of the stall as usual, and he was ready for her visit. Sara stepped inside the stall, unhooked the IV set, placed the plug in the catheter in Quincy's neck, and snapped the lead rope on Quincy's halter.

"You ready to try this boy?"

He just stared at her as if to say, "Let's go."

Chapter 26

Sara opened the stall door and led Quincy out. He was unsteady at first, but when they turned the corner, and he saw the open roll up door leading to the outside, his gait quickened, and he became steadier on his feet. He was pulling Sara by the time they got outside.

Sara walked Quincy to the turn out area, unsnapped the lead rope, and let him loose in the round pen. At first, Quincy just took a few steps and sniffed around to check out his new environment, but then, to Sara's surprise, he started slowly trotting around the pen.

"Whoa, Quincy, whoa!!" Sara screamed. He sure didn't need to be trotting. He might feel better, but his body was still in pretty bad shape. Quincy stopped at Sara's command. She started walking to him to snap the lead rope back into place. She couldn't let him loose. She would have to hand walk and graze him.

As Sara approached, Quincy stepped back. She took another step. He took another step back. She told him to whoa as she took a step toward him. He took a step back. He was playing a game - a game, which involved him not getting caught.

"Great, Quincy," Sara berated the horse. "I bring you out here to enjoy yourself, you overdo it, and now I try to catch you, and you aren't going to let me. Don't make me go in and find someone to help me catch you. Now, please come here." Sara begged.

Sara took another step toward Quincy, and as if the horse understood, he let Sara catch him. After she got the lead rope back on the halter, Quincy placed his head again on Sara's shoulder to try and butter her up.

"You're killing me, fella'. You do that head thing way too much, but you know what you're doing, don't you? You're making me love you. That's what you're doing. Now, come on. I'm going to walk you around, let you graze some, and then we're going back inside, understand?" Sara asked Quincy.

He understood. Sara and Quincy exited the round pen and went out to the grass. Sara let him graze awhile, and then she would walk him a couple of steps, and let him graze some more. After ten minutes or so, Quincy seemed content to just graze, so Sara plopped down beside him and loosely held the lead.

Sara knew sitting down beside a horse wasn't the smartest idea in the world, but what could she say, she trusted Quincy. As Quincy picked at the grass, Sara began to look for a four-leaf clover, a habit she had since she was a child. The sun was bright. A small breeze was blowing and the sky was a brilliant blue.

Sara could hear the traffic on Neyland, but she blocked those noises out. The knot in her stomach had begun to subside earlier, and now, it was gone. Sitting here beside Quincy, listening to the leaves in the trees rustle in the wind, Sara began to relax. The sun warming her back and the sound of Quincy munching grass was putting Sara at ease.

They stayed like that for a while. Sara sitting cross-legged in the lawn with her head down picking through the grass and Quincy, one leg in front of the other bending down to enjoy his afternoon snack.

Sara had many afternoons like this one before at home. When she was younger, as soon as she got home from school, she was off to the barn. Most of the time, she wouldn't even saddle her horse. Dan would be waiting for her.

They would stand in the hall of the barn. Sara would get the old stump out of the tack room. She would put the bridle on her horse, Dan, and lead him up to the stump. He would stand while she stepped up on the stump and then crawled onto his back, and off they would go.

Behind her parent's barn, there were two fields with a creek in between. Beyond the fields, there were miles and miles of woods. Sara's father had made several trails through these woods. The trails led to other fields and other woods. Sara would ride for hours there.

Those afternoon rides took Sara away from all worries. It was if she and Dan were one, with one mind, and moving with one motion. Dan knew the trail as well as Sara did and most of the time, she would barely have to hold the reins. They would ride through the trail in the woods with the leaves from overburdened branches tickling Sara on the shoulder and face.

Sara could remember how the wind would blow through the trees then softly kiss her face and hair. The trees were dense. Small pinpoints of sunlight would break through dancing on the trail. The only sounds would be the birds singing in the trees and maybe a rabbit or squirrel scurrying to their hiding place.

She and Dan would arrive at the first field, on a hill, past the woods. He would walk into the middle of the field. He would stop there because they both knew the routine. She would slide off his back, sit down in the grass, and let him drop his head and graze while she looked for four leaf clovers or just gazed down the hill at the farmland below. She could see her home and watch as her mother hung out clothes on the line or as her sister practiced softball in the back yard.

When she and Dan were ready to go back, Sara would find the old gate to a half torn down fence at the edge of the field. She'd climb up on the fence, and Dan would stand for her to hop on his back. Sometimes, they would just turn and go back home. Sometimes, they would ride farther. It depended on the day, Sara's and Dan's mood, and how many chores or how much homework she had waiting on her at home.

Some days, Sara would find that four leaf clover in the pasture at the top of the hill. She wasn't superstitious and didn't believe in luck so much, but it always seemed the rest of the day somehow was easier if she had a four-leaf clover in her hand when she climbed back up on Dan.

Today, with Quincy grazing right beside her, much the same way Dan had always done, Sara saw the treasure in the grass. The four-leaf clover was hidden in the grass right below her boot. She plucked the clover, looked up at Quincy, and smiled.

"It's a sign, fella. Everything's going to be okay."

Chapter 27

Even with the luck of the four-leaf clover, Sara didn't get to go home before Quincy's eight o'clock treatment. She had decided to stay and get everything ready for Dino and Thumper's departure tomorrow. She called their owners to let them know when to pick them up, and she also called Mrs. Taylor to let her know how Quincy did on his little romp outside. She treated Quincy and got him ready for the night.

Sara left the clinic around eight thirty, let Jake out, and now, both she and Jake were resting on the couch watching some television. It was nice to watch the mind-numbing device and relax. A pretty interesting crime show was playing, and Sara was just thankful she could find something besides reality shows. She had enough reality in her own life.

As the crime show came to an end and the brilliant detective finally caught the perpetrator, Sara found herself yawning and her eyes closing. It was time to go to bed. If she went to bed now, she would have exactly four hours of sleep before it was time to get up and treat Quincy again. That should make for a cozy little nap.

Sara offered Jake another chance to go outside, and the pup declined. He was also ready to get a nap. As Sara climbed into bed and hoisted Jake up on the pillow beside her, she kissed the pup goodnight, and within minutes, she was in a much-needed deep and peaceful sleep, but then she began to dream.

Sara was again standing at the riverbank with the water threatening to rise and flood. There was no peace before the storm this time. The thunderstorm was in full rage as Sara stood looking to the other side. This time in her dream, the horses were far off, but she could see them getting closer. They had first appeared as fuzzy grey dots in the distance, and the torrential rain made those dots fade in and out, but one thing was sure, the dots were getting larger and closer with each minute.

"I just need to stand here. I don't need to try and get under the trees or get under some cover. If I don't move, I won't fall into the water, and if I don't fall into the water, I won't be carried to the other side." Sara thought to herself knowing full well that if she was carried to the other side that the distant moving band of horses would be upon her as soon as she surfaced from the water.

A lightning bolt tore from the sky and hit one of the trees behind Sara with a deafening peal of thunder following. Sparks flew from the tree as the tree began a downward descent to the earth - a descent that would land the bulk of the massive tree on top of Sara. She had to move. She had no choice, and she had to move now.

Sara lunged to her side and landed on a small clump of land that had turned to mud with all the rain. The mud was slick, and against all her best efforts, she began to slide. As she fell, her body lurched toward the riverbank and began to roll and slip closer and closer to the water. Sara was trying to grab anything she could to keep her up on the bank, but everything she grabbed came loose from the mud-soaked soil. She was going to go into the water, and there was absolutely nothing she could do about it.

Sara knew this was a dream even as she was dreaming it, but knowing that did not make her heart beat any slower or her struggle any less as the current began sweeping her to the other side of the bank. She did not want to see those front hooves of the leader coming down on her skull. She did not want to feel as if she was drowning in the water before her body rose to take a ragged breath only to be pulled under once again. She demanded herself to wake up. Her mind would not obey.

She opened her eyes as she surfaced the raging waters knowing what she would see on the other side of the bank. The horses were there, and their leader, in all his fierce grace, was waiting on the other side for her. The current took her down again. She could tell she was not moving down river but across river just as she had in her first dream. She surfaced again.

He was there, shaking his head up and down, his front hoof pulverizing the muddy ground with impatience each time he pawed. His loud roaring call belted through the storm, the rain, and the thunder. He was ready for Sara to appear on the other side, so he could finish her once and for all.

Sara was suffocating under the water, and the instinctual need for air won its battle against her fear. She surfaced, and not surprised in the least, she was now on the other bank looking up at the leader rise on his powerful back legs to aim those front hooves at Sara's skull. She was wet, cold, and scared. She couldn't think or reason. She could only watch, as if in slow motion, the hooves began to descend from the stormy air.

Pieces of mud and slime were caked to the underbelly and front legs of the leader from pawing the earth. The hooves which would soon crack Sara's skull were caked with mud as the falling rain rolled off the edges of the ragged hooves onto the ground. She felt the first one descend and hit its target. The pain was like a searing hot iron running from the top of her head through her spine. She began to scream in short, ragged breaths.

The alarm clock was going off in cadence with her screams as Sara woke in the dark night. Jake was there licking her about her face and ears. The covers were off the bed and sweat covered her body. Jake was trembling. He wasn't sure what she had been dreaming, but her moans had awakened him and the smell of fear surrounded her. He just wanted her to wake up.

"It's okay, Buddy. It was just another bad dream - a really bad dream." Sara stroked Jake and rubbed his little ears to console him. The pup saw she was awake and okay and immediately calmed down.

"Gotta' get ready, Jake. We gotta' go treat Quincy."

Back into the night Sara and Jake went. Knoxville was quiet at two o'clock in the morning, even on Kingston Pike. Jake and Sara had no trouble navigating their way to the large animal clinic. As Sara climbed out of the truck, she swooped Jake up in her arms. There weren't many here tonight. No reason for him to sit out here by himself.

Sara let Jake down as soon as they got into the clinic. This wasn't the little puppy's first visit to the large animal clinic. Sara planned on taking Jake with her on farm calls once she started practice. He probably wouldn't get out at a lot of those calls, but he needed to know his way around animals any way.

She tried to take him around animals and other people any time the opportunity presented itself. Sara had picked a blue heeler in part because of their legendary loyalty and protection regarding their owner. She also needed a dog that had a natural instinct around animals and that her clients would not mind being on their farm. She felt blue heelers fit the bill, and Jake fit the bill perfectly.

As Sara made her way to Quincy's stall, Jake followed in perfect step beside her. He had been down here enough for Sara to teach him to stay beside her and not to run off and explore the new surroundings. He was at attention because his nose as well as his ears told him that cows and horses were around, and he hoped he might have to jump into action at any time. Sara looked down at the puppy and laughed.

"You're ready to bite some heels at any moment, aren't you, Jake? I don't think we'll need your services tonight, but you stay here close to me just in case I do."

Chapter 28

Quincy had heard Sara and Jake as they were approaching and gave the appropriate whinny to say hello.

"Jake, come here, I want you to meet someone," Sara commanded.

"Now, sit, Jake."

Jake sat at the front of Quincy's stall on command and looked up at what must have seemed like, to him, a gigantic horse. Quincy had Jake's full attention and his little plump body shook with anticipation.

"Okay, now, Quincy, you say hi to Jake."

On cue, Quincy lowered his head through the opening in the stall door. Because of the door, Quincy could only lower his head about a foot from where Jake sat.

The big horse looked at the little puppy and the little puppy looked at the big horse. Both were using their noses to figure out what the other was, and then, before Sara could stop him, Jake jumped into the air and nipped Quincy playfully on the nose.

Quincy pulled his head back into the stall and shook his nose. Jake wanted to play, but Quincy wasn't interested. He thought the puppy was amusing, and he would be happy to watch the little thing jump and scurry around - as long as it stayed out of his stall and away from his nose.

"Okay, Jake, no more horsing around tonight. Doesn't look like Quincy likes nips on the nose, and I don't blame him. Come over here, and I'll get Quincy's meds ready." Sara walked to the treatment station by Quincy's stall. Jake followed.

"Sit, Jake, now stay." The puppy obeyed.

Jake sat waiting as Sara treated Quincy. Quincy seemed to be improving every time Sara treated him. His breathing was getting better as well as his appetite and attitude. Sara was very hopeful. In less than forty-eight hours, Quincy had improved tremendously.

The treatment, as always, went off without a hitch, and as Sara exited the stall, Quincy whinnied low.

"What is it, Quincy?" Sara asked.

She turned back to face him. He walked over and nudged Sara.

"You want a good night scratch? Is that it?"

Sara scratched Quincy under the jaw and stroked his head and neck. He sidled up right beside her and gently leaned into her to let her know his approval.

"I can't do this all night, Quincy. I need sleep, and in case you've forgotten, there's a little ball of fur out there that won't stand for this long."

Quincy leaned into Sara for just a moment longer, and then he stepped back, turned, and walked to the back of his stall.

"Okay, I guess that's enough for now, huh? I'll be back in the morning. I'll try to get here early so we can take a walk and let you graze. Is that a deal?"

Quincy stood watching Sara as she left the stall. She took used needles and syringes to the work station and disposed of them and put the other equipment back in its place. She and Jake proceeded to head toward the exit door. Sara turned to look at her patient.

Quincy had walked to the front of the stall and was standing, with his big head out the stall door, watching her walk away. Sara felt a strong tug at her heart. She waved goodbye to Quincy as she turned the corner, and she and Jake, paddling quietly beside her, went out into the parking lot and home.

Sara fell asleep as soon as her head hit the pillow. She and Jake slept soundly for the rest of the night.

Chapter 29

When Sara arrived at the clinic the next morning, Quincy almost looked like a normal horse. The wheezing was gone, and she had to look closely at his chest to notice any increased effort in his breathing. His temperature was normal and his lungs sounded much better. Sara was very pleased.

Sara gave Quincy his morning feed and while he was munching away, went and got his meds. He never looked up when she gave the IV meds into the port, and she was surprised that he was a little stubborn in taking his breathing treatment. He really didn't want to spend that time away from his morning meal, which, again, was a good sign.

After the breathing treatment was over, Quincy went right back to his food, and Sara stood beside him for a moment stroking his beautiful, long neck. If he kept on improving, he could easily go home in a couple of days.

"You're a lot better, Son. Judy would be very proud. She told me you were a fighter, and she was right. I can almost see the horse you used to be, and that musta' been some kind of horse."

Sara continued to stroke the horses head and neck as he ate. The familiar smell of the barn and horses, the repetitive motion of stroking his neck, and her patient's obvious improvement, brought Sara a peace she hadn't felt in days.

For nearly three days, the most sleep Sara had gotten had been at three and four hour intervals. With little sleep and not much more to eat, Sara was tired, and she was beginning to wear down. She felt as if she were walking in a haze with her nerve endings humming most of the time and a lead brick in her stomach. Standing there, with Quincy, she felt calm. He was doing better - it was all worth it.

Sara continued to rub Quincy for a couple more minutes and soak up the feeling that all was well. She glanced down at her watch and knew she had to get busy if she planned on taking him for a walk this morning after he ate.

"Okay, Buddy. I'm going to run down to the break room, get some coffee, and call Judy to let her know how you're doing. I'll be back in a minute to let you out, sound good?" Sara asked Quincy.

He never raised his head. He was too intent on his morning meal. Sara gave him one last pat and headed off for coffee.

Hillary was already in the break room and on her second cup of coffee. Sara could tell she had some news by the look on her face.

"What's going on?" asked Sara.

"Well, you know how me and you complained about not being able to go to Ames because our large animal rotations didn't work out?"

"Yeah...."

"Dr. Butler just came through and told me they are going to have to go to Ames this weekend for a special trip. You can sign up at the large animal reception desk. They are going to draw names from our rotation, the large animal surgery rotation, and radiology. Isn't that great?!"

"You're kidding me!!!" Sara exclaimed. Sara had heard about the famous Ames Plantation trips from her vets at home and from some of the upper classmates when they had been in clinics. She and Hillary had not been considered for the trips this year because they had been in small animal rotations when the trips were taken. She couldn't believe their luck.

Ames Plantation was a historic plantation in West Tennessee. The trips usually lasted a couple of days. During their stay, the students were able to work on the animals that lived at Ames and this included horses, cows, and pigs. Students got to stay in the dorms provided at Ames and the plantation hosts provided all meals. The work, the rooms, and the food were almost legendary.

Everyone that wanted to go into large animal practice wanted to go to Ames for the experience to work on the different agricultural animals. Most students that didn't want to go into large animal practice still wanted to go to Ames Plantation because of all the stories about the homemade meals and the beautiful scenery.

Dr. Butler, a long-time large animal clinician and professor, always took the group, and he was well known for his patience and his sense of humor. Sara had already been on some ambulatory calls with him and several day trips to the state's dairies and beef cattle operations. He was hilarious, had great stories, and pretty much let the students run the show as long as they were doing everything right. He would be a wonderful mentor on the Ames trip.

If Hillary and Sara were really lucky, they might both get to go. Both girls had huge smiles on their faces and then suddenly, Sara's smile faded as she thought of the only reason she didn't need to go to Ames - Quincy.

"Wait a minute - I know what you're thinking. I know that look on your face. Someone else can take care of Quincy, and besides, he's getting better." Hillary almost whined.

"I know, I know. He looks really good this morning. Did you say we are leaving day after tomorrow?" Sara asked.

"Yeah, but you have to sign up today. They are going to draw the names this afternoon. Come on, Sara; if your name gets drawn and he gets worse, you could always back out. There'll be plenty of people who would want your spot. At least sign up."

"I gotta' make sure Leanne can take care of Jake, too, though."

"You know Leanne is going to take care of Jake, and if she can't, you can board him here. I don't see that as a problem at all. The only possible problem I see is you not letting someone else take care of Quincy."

"If he keeps on improving, he should be ready to go home the day we go to Ames, and you're right, if he gets worse, I can always get someone else to take my place on the Ames trip. I'm going to grab some coffee, go sign up, and then find Leanne."

"Sounds good to me."

The girls gave each other a high-five as Sara left the room with coffee in hand on the way to reception. The list to Ames only had a few names on it. At the bottom of the list, in bold letters, was written - only three get to go. Sara sure hoped she was going to be one of them.

Chapter 30

Sara left reception and started down the hall toward the food animal ward. She knew Leanne would be doing her morning treatments. She also knew that Leanne would not sign up for Ames because she would not want to leave Bubbles.

Sara knew she would probably feel the same way about Jake when he got to be an old man, but right now, she figured he would be fine without her for a weekend. She also knew he would be in good hands with Leanne.

It didn't take Sara long to find her. Leanne was working on a baby calf whose mother had tried to kill it shortly after birth. The calf had to have surgery yesterday because of the wounds it's mother inflicted, but looked to be pretty spry today. Leanne was bottle-feeding the calf.

As far as Sara was concerned, there was nothing much sweeter than seeing a baby calf or baby foal suckling the bottle. Everyone had much prefer they be suckling their mother, but sometimes it just didn't work out that way.

"Little guy doing okay?" Sara asked.

"He's running a little fever this morning but looks like he's rebounding pretty good. If he takes his bottle well today and his temp is down tomorrow, we'll probably send him home. His mother did a pretty good job on him, though."

"Momma a first-timer?"

"Yeah, she's a heifer. Don't know that they'll keep her, but she's supposed to be a high-priced heifer, so they probably will. If she tries to kill her second, though, I figure she'll be gone."

"Glad we're breeding animals with such good dispositions." Sara laughed sarcastically. Leanne shook her head and rolled her eyes in agreement.

"So, what's got you on the food animal side? Gotta patient over here?"

"No, I need to ask you a favor but I need to ask you a question first."

"Okay."

"You planning on putting your name in on the drawing for Ames."

"I thought about it, but I don't want to leave Bubbles. She's too old and that would upset her too much."

"That's kinda' what I thought you'd say."

"You need someone to look after Jake in case your name does get drawn?"

"How'd you guess?"

"I just know how bad you wanted to go, and now you have the chance. I also figure that horse of yours is doing better or you wouldn't ask, right?"

"Yeah, he's doing a lot better. I'm hoping by the time I go to Ames, he'll be going home."

"I sure hope so, Sara. I'm glad he's doing better. Just let me know this afternoon if your name gets drawn. I'll take care of the little pup for you."

"Thanks, Leanne."

"No problem."

The girls watched in silence as the calf finished his bottle. He pulled on the nipple a couple of more times to make sure no more milk was there. Leanne finally had to pull it from his mouth. He was a cute little bugger, but Sara had stayed as long as she could.

"I'll let you know." Sara told Leanne as she turned to go down to Quincy's stall for his morning turnout. She would stop at the phone on the way to call Mrs. Taylor.

"See ya' later, Sara." Leanne waved goodbye.

Chapter 31

There was a phone in the hall close to Quincy's stall, and Sara knew Mrs. Taylor's number by heart. Judy Taylor picked up the phone on the first ring and was thrilled with the news that Quincy was much better. She asked Sara when he could come home, and Sara let her know they would still need to watch him to make sure the new medications were doing their job, but maybe, hopefully, he would be able to go home within the next 48 hours. Judy squealed on the other end of the phone with delight. Sara laughed, told Mrs. Taylor she would be calling her tonight, and hung up the phone.

On cue, Quincy stuck his head out of the stall down the hall.

"Okay, guy, let's go." Sara grabbed Quincy's lead rope from the stall, clipped his halter, plugged his IV, and off they went toward those rolled up double doors. Quincy was actually prancing to get outside. Sara smiled a wide smile and cooed to Quincy to slow him down.

Once outside, Sara walked Quincy for a couple of minutes and then led him to the same small patch of grass. The grass was too wet with dew for Sara to sit down this morning, but not to wet for Quincy to graze with vigor. Sara stood and looked out at the morning.

The morning air had a bite that reminded one that spring wasn't quite here, but you could tell it was coming. Since Knoxville was only an hour or so away from the Great Smoky Mountains, the air also had a clean, fresh smell that most small cities did not have. Knoxville was funny that way. It was a small city, but most of the time, it had a small town atmosphere, and it was gorgeous. From the campus of the University of Tennessee to West End to Chapman Highway, Knoxville had a definite charm, and Sara would hate to leave it, but she would after graduation.

She was headed back to West Tennessee. Knoxville with its history and its dogwoods and the life she had here would always hold a special place in her heart, but she was ready to get on with living. She was ready to be "grown," and that meant moving, starting her career and getting ready for whatever else life had in store for her down the road. Either way, she would miss this town.

"Isn't it funny, Qunicy? When I start practice, I won't be more than a couple of hours away from you. I might even come down to Memphis and visit you sometime if Judy doesn't mind. Whatta' you think?"

Quincy never looked up. He just flicked one of his big ears at her to let her know he was listening and kept grazing. He was enjoying this time outside and so was Sara, even if it was a little chilly. Sara glanced at her watched and realized she had been lost in her own thoughts for some time. They still had a couple of minutes before she had to take Quincy back in to be on time for morning rounds. She let the big boy graze and enjoyed the morning.

Chapter 32

Dr. Summers and the crew went through morning rounds easily. The rotation and especially Sara had been blessed with many outpatients in the last few days. That meant most of the patients had been seen and then gone home. There were few hospitalized patients, and as had been their practice over the last several days, the last hospitalized patient to see was Quincy.

Julia was surprised and somewhat pleased with the horses' condition. Unbeknownst to Sara, Julia had laid both a hand and an eye on this horse several times since he had been in their care. Julia could tell Sara had been taking wonderful care of Quincy, and from all appearances, he was doing well. Julia was pleased with the horses' condition, but she was also pleased for Sara. She knew from personal experience the satisfaction that came from pouring your heart into a patient and seeing that patient improve day by day.

Julia also knew that Judy would be more than pleased. Sara, and most of her classmates, did not have the experience yet to know that as a veterinarian, you work for the animal, but you also work for the owner and especially if the owner loves the animal. Veterinary medicine isn't just about the animal - it's about the owner, too.

Great satisfaction comes from healing - healing the animal and healing the owner's heart and sometimes, their soul. Julia knew Sara would see a perfect example of this the day she discharged Quincy back into Judy's care. It was a wonderful part of the actual practice of being a veterinarian.

"So, your boy looks good, Sara. Any updates?" asked Julia.

"He's eating well, temperature is normal, lungs sound much better, other vitals are normal and he is feeling good. I think maybe we can discontinue the IV fluids and just leave the catheter in for the medicine, do some more bloodwork tomorrow to make sure that's looking better, and if it is and he continues to improve, go home the next day. What do you think, Dr. Summers?"

"I think you're right on the money, Sara. Continue with the iv medications and fluids through today, we'll do bloodwork tomorrow and see how that's going and of course, continue with the breathing treatments. He looks good. Good job, Sara."

"Thanks, Dr. Summers." Sara smiled a quiet smile of satisfaction.

"Okay, guys, now let's talk about today." Julia told the group changing from Quincy to the day's work ahead. "I need Hillary and Sara to go out on ambulatory today, and I need Jessica, Doug, and Josh to stay with me here in the clinics and see some incoming patients."

"Sara - you and Hillary get on over to the ambulatory bays. I think Dr. Rodriquez is waiting for you there. The rest of you guys follow me." Julia turned and left with the rest of the students. Sara and Hillary headed to the ambulatory trucks. Both girls were amazed that Dr. Summers had put them together again.

"Beautiful day to be outside, Sara. Dr. Summers must be getting soft here at the end of the rotation - letting us do stuff together." Hillary said to Sara.

"Guess so, or maybe she knows we work together well as a team, and with Dr. Rodriquez, the help of a team is definitely needed." Sara giggled.

"Well, it is a beautiful day, and maybe if Dr. Rodriquez isn't too intense today, we can get him to tell us about Ames."

"It is a beautiful day, but I wouldn't count on Dr. Rodriquez not being intense. You look up the word in the dictionary, and his picture's beside it." Sara replied.

Both girls were shaking their heads and laughing all the way to the trucks.

Chapter 33

In veterinary medicine, ambulatory service doesn't mean what most people think. It doesn't mean, necessarily that there is an emergency somewhere or that you ride in an animal ambulance with sirens blasting at ninety miles per hour. Ambulatory really just means to be able to move or moving, and being on the ambulatory rotation basically meant you rode around, in a regular veterinary truck, and did farm calls. Sometimes there were emergencies, but it was mostly just regular, run-of-the mill, farm calls like vaccinating, deworming, looking at a couple of sick or hurt animals, and helping farmers manage their herds.

Also, in veterinary medicine, a farm truck might not mean what most people think it means. A farm truck at the University of Tennessee College of Veterinary Medicine consisted of a double cab truck with a vet box in back. This vet box was plugged up or charged up every night upon arrival at the large animal clinic so the water and power sources would be available for the next day's work. When you went out on a farm call, you had plenty of running water and power available right at your fingertips, if needed. These vet boxes were also stocked with everything a farm veterinarian needed. They were like little mobile veterinary clinics, and ambulatory was always fun.

Well, mostly fun - as long as you didn't get Dr. Rodriquez, or that was what Sara had heard from some of her classmates. Dr. Butler was always fun, and usually the other ambulatory clinician, Dr. Hopkins, was also a blast. Everyone agreed on those two, but Dr. Rodriquez had a mixed reputation. He had a reputation of being impatient and intense.

Dr. Rodriquez got the reputation of being impatient and intense because he was impatient and intense. He was from Puerto Rico and spoke English with a very pronounced Spanish accent. He was around 6'2, muscular, with piercing dark brown eyes, jet-black hair and a goatee. In every right, he should have been a very attractive man but God had played around with his forehead and his nose.

God had made these features in some way that just intensified Dr. Rodriquez's intenseness, if that made any sense. He was, in all actuality, kinda' scary looking, and Sara could easily remember the first time she had to go on ambulatory with him. She had been nearly scared to death.

During the first session, Sara had been with two of her classmates. Instead of the usual discussions about clinics or diseases or cases or even light-hearted bantering between classmates, the four of them had ridden in complete silence the whole day until they came to the farms. When they got out at the farms, Dr. Rodriquez would tell them why they were there, ask them a few questions, and then watch them work or have them watch him work.

When they were done, they would all pile back into the truck and ride in complete silence until they came to another farm. The tense silence would only be broken if another motorist did something Dr. Rodriquez did not like. There would be a stream of what Sara thought was probably Spanish profanity flow from Dr. Rodriquez's lips and then, again, silence.

When Sara got out of the truck that first long day, she hoped she would never ride with Dr. Rodriquez again - but she did, and not only did she have to ride with him on ambulatory, she had him for part of her large animal surgery rotation, too. She learned, to her dismay, that Dr. Rodriquez was intense, but not in the way she had thought. He was intense about his career, about being a good veterinarian, about teaching students who cared about veterinary medicine, and about life, in general.

He was also impatient - impatient with people who didn't care for their animals like he knew animals should be cared for. He was impatient with students who were lazy and didn't care to learn and didn't do their jobs. He was impatient with university politics that demanded certain things from him that he didn't feel were important at all, and he was impatient with himself if he felt he did not do a good job.

He was not impatient, however, if he could tell that you did really care about the animals you treated. He was not impatient if he found out that you were interested in horses and cows and you wanted to learn as much about them as you could, and actually, Sara had found that he did have some soft spots, and deep down, under that somewhat fascinating but scary outward appearance, he could be kind and could be fun and had a very sarcastic, witty sense of humor.

Today, unlike the first day Sara went on ambulatory with Dr. Rodriquez, she found she couldn't wait to get in the truck and out into the beautiful day. Dr. Rodriquez, Hillary, and she would have a good day. He would teach them, he would quiz them, but at the end of the day, they would all work together and by the time they got back to the large animal hospital, they would be laughing and joking about something. Sara just didn't know what yet.

Chapter 34

"Ladies, let's hurry and get in the truck. Our first call sounds like a colicky horse. Let's get moving" Dr. Rodriquez called out to Hillary and Sara.

A horse with colic is not like a baby with colic. A horse with colic can be a very serious thing. It is true that with colic, the baby and the horse, have a bellyache, but that's probably where most of the similarities stop. First of all, a horse, on average, usually weighs around a thousand pounds - a thousand pounds of muscle. So, when a baby cries, screams, writhes, and throws a fit with colic, the parents usually soothe that baby and can get it back to sleep.

When a thousand pound animal writhes, rolls, gets up and immediately falls back down, you can't put it in your arms and soothe it down. Some horses with colic can be so violent that it is hard to get near them to treat them and still stay physically safe.

The second thing about a horse with colic is that colic can kill a horse. Parents might think their baby with colic is probably going to kill them from sleep deprivation, but a horse can die from colic. Sometimes part of their fifty to seventy feet of small intestines twist, sometimes the flexure in their colon gets some type of blockage that won't move. Horses can't vomit and enemas hardly ever work on a colic horse.

About eighty percent of colics can be handled with pain medications, some medications by mouth, and intravenous fluids. The remaining twenty percent can be nightmares and require surgery. Surgery for colic is very costly. Needless to say, all horses that need surgery don't get it.

Knowing this, Hillary and Sara didn't take their time getting in the truck. They loaded into the truck quickly and prepared to go. Dr. Rodriquez started the truck and sped out onto the highway.

"Where's the horse, Dr. Rodriquez?" Hillary asked.

"It's about 20 miles down Chapman Highway. They called about five minutes ago and said the mare seemed pretty bad. She's about eight months bred, so she might just be uncomfortable from the foal, but they say she's up and down a lot and won't eat her food or graze. The owners found her about thirty minutes ago."

"Have they given her anything yet?" Sara piped in.

"No, they don't have anything on hand at the barn. I talked to them and told them to walk her to try to keep her up, and we'd be there as soon as we could."

The way Dr. Rodriquez drove, it wouldn't take them long to get there. On the drive, he asked Hillary and Sara some questions about colic like causes, medical treatments, how one knew surgery was needed, and prognosis with colic. They were driving up the driveway before either student barely had time to know they were there.

As they topped the drive, the house was off to the left but they saw the wife standing, waiting by the gate that opened to the pastures and the barn. As she opened the gate, she motioned to the back of the barn. Dr. Rodriquez drove through with a nod, and they headed toward the back.

The husband was walking an obviously pregnant mare. The mare would stop, try to lie down from the pain, but the husband was able to push her forward. Dr. Rodriquez, Sara, and Hillary got out and started to work.

The students had been with Dr. Rodriquez enough to know that the condition the mare was in meant he would examine her immediately. This appeared to be an emergency situation, so there would be no examination by the students, discussions, and then treatment. He would go first and then he would tell Hillary and Sara what to do.

As Dr. Rodriquez spoke to the owners and started examining the mare, Hillary and Sara went to the back of the truck and got all the meds and equipment they would need to treat this mare. This included a shot for the pain, sedation, the nasogastric tube, the laxative diluted with a gallon of water they poured in the stainless, steel bucket, another gallon of plain water, a pump, a rectal sleeve, a thermometer, a twitch and lube. Dr. Rodriquez had his stethoscope in his pocket.

By the time they got to the horse, Dr. Rodriquez was close to the end of his examination. He turned to the girls and started his orders.

"Thermometer." He took the mare's rectal temperature. Horses' don't really care for a thermometer in their mouth.

"Her temp is normal." Dr. Rodriquez reported. "Now hand me sleeve and need some lube."

He put the long plastic sleeve that covered his right hand and most of his right arm on. He held out his arm, and Sara poured the lube on the sleeve. He inserted his whole arm into the mare's rectum to feel her colon and possibly small intestines to try and find a blockage or a twist. The mare didn't seem to mind very much. She just wanted the pain in her belly to stop.

"Okay, give the banamine, and I also want her to have some torbugesic, Hillary." These were the pain meds and the sedation.

"Sara," Dr. Rodriquez commanded, "you get to tube her."

Uggghhhh, Sara thought. She had tubed a horse about five times so far in clinics, so she was not an expert by any means, but she definitely needed the practice. Dr. Rodriquez would not be there to help her in a couple of months. She needed to get good at this procedure.

When a horse colicked, tubing it was standard practice. The veterinarian put a large, soft plastic tube into the horse's nostril and basically passed it from there, down the esophagus and into the stomach. Because of the horse's anatomy, it could not be passed through the long mouth and teeth.

On most horses, you could even see the tube through the neck as it went down the esophagus once they decided to swallow. If a horse didn't decide to swallow, the tube could go into the trachea and down into the lungs.

Once you started pumping fluid into the tube, you better be sure the tube was in the stomach and not the lungs because if it were in the lungs, you would kill the horse by drowning it. If you put too much pressure on the tube trying to pass it, you could also bump the sinuses in the nose enough to make them bleed.

If the horse moved it's head and fought a lot while you were trying to pass the tube, you could also make them bleed. The horse didn't bleed a drop or two if these things happened. It looked like a gallon of blood streaming out their noses. The owners always loved that.

In one way, tubing a horse was a pretty simple procedure, but in some ways, it could really be difficult.

Hillary had given the meds in the vein to the horse, and the mare looked like she was already getting some relief. Sara walked to the front of the mare and started putting on the twitch. The mare resisted, and Sara didn't really blame her, but she knew that if she fought her on this, she would definitely need the twitch when she went to tube her.

The twitch, to some, might seem inhumane. It is usually a rope that is attached to a long piece of wood or pipe. The rope goes around the horse's nose and then the piece of wood or pipe is twisted to twist the rope tightly around the horse's nose. Sara even thought it was bordering on brutal until she worked at the vet clinic at home.

Time after time, Sara saw the twitch go on the horse's nose when something medical was done to them. She finally asked one of the veterinarian's there why it had to be done. He had been a veterinarian for over twenty years and worked mostly on horses.

"It just works better for the horse and for us. You've learned in vet school how when the twitch is applied, it releases natural endorphins to the horse, so first of all, I think they feel less pain when we have to do something to them, and usually, not always, but usually, it calms them down." He told Sara.

"Second of all, Sara," he continued, "I've learned that I get hurt a lot less and can do my job a lot faster with that twitch. When you've gotten kicked and pawed a couple of times, you'll realize that's it's best for the horse and you. You can't treat all the other horses that need help if you are lying in a hospital bed." He said and smiled.

About two weeks after that, Sara had been holding the twitch on a horse that he was tubing just as she was about to this mare. She had seen this 6 foot 6 inch big man fly through the air about the same time her foot went completely numb. The horse, even though it was twitched, had struck out with one of its front legs and pawed with such force that he had flown back and had stomped her foot in the process.

It was so quick, she never even seen the strike, just the after effects. The vet had rolled, paused a minute on the ground, and dusted himself off. She tightened the twitch harder, and they tubed the horse without another problem. She could barely take her boot off that night because her foot was so swollen. The incident had taught her a valuable lesson.

Sara returned her thoughts to the mare at hand, took a deep breath, looked at Hillary and nodded at her to hold the halter tight and grab an ear. This time, the mare let her twitch her. First, Sara had to get the tube started. She dipped the end of the tube that would go in the horse's nose in the water so it would be lubricated and put the other end of the long tube in her mouth.

She stood slightly to the side of the mare, so in case the mare did paw, she would not get the full force of it. She began to slowly advance the tube up the nostril until she got to the point where she felt the mare's epiglottis. She carefully prodded the epiglottis with the tube to make the mare swallow, and she did.

Once the mare swallowed, Sara blew on her end of the tube to help the esophagus dilate and allow the tube to more easily descend down into the stomach. The blowing also helped her visualize the air in the esophagus to let her know she was in the right place. If you blew on the tube, and the tube was in the esophagus, then you could see the flow of air going down the left side of the horse's neck.

Sara saw the flutter on the left side of the mare's neck. She advanced the tube some more until most of the tube was in the mare. Sara blew on the tube once more and then took her mouth off the tube. Gas bubbled up through the tube and Sara could smell grass. She knew she was in the stomach.

She looked over to Hillary and nodded. Hillary brought the bucket with only water. The pump was already in the bucket. Hillary held the bucket as Sara attached the tube to the pump. She pumped some water through the tube, disconnected the tube from the pump and waited to see what would happen. They were refluxing the mare.

Horses cannot vomit. So, if their stomachs are bloated from a blockage high up in the small intestines, the stomach will swell. When a tube is placed in the stomach and water is pumped in, it almost acts as a valve for pressure release. Stomach contents can, at times, come back up the tube with such force that a veterinarian can easily get splattered with them or if they are unfortunate enough to have their mouth on the tube, get a mouthful of horse stomach contents.

Sara was grateful that neither happened with this mare. They pumped water several different times and when no reflux came back up, Sara signaled Hillary that it was time for the laxative. If they had reflux, they would not have used the laxative because it would have only gone to the stomach and no further because of a blockage high in the gastrointestinal system.

Hillary changed the buckets, Sara attached the tube to the pump, and then they pumped a gallon of laxative into the mare. Sara then took the tube and pulled it from the mare. They had successfully tubed the horse. Dr. Rodriquez had been on standby the whole time but had not had to help or utter a word. Now, he did.

"Okay, ladies, I want you to examine the horse and let me know what you find while the owners and I step over here and talk about her condition."

It took them approximately 15 minutes to examine the mare. Her heart rate was slightly above normal due to the pain. Her gums were good and pink. Her respiration was normal, and her gut sounds were slow which was to be expected with colic. She was already feeling better and not wanting to lie down. Her temperature was normal. The students finished the exam. Hillary held the mare while Sara walked over to Dr. Rodriquez.

"Watch her closely for the next twenty-four hours. She seems like she already feels better." He said to the owners and pointed to the mare. She was already trying to graze. "If you need us, call us."

He nodded to the owners who expressed their thanks, collected his fee, and started walking back to the truck. The students followed.

When they got back to the truck, they discussed the mare and her chances. Dr. Rodriquez had not felt any impaction or enlarged intestines when he palpated the mare. She had quickly gone back to grazing with the pain medication and the laxatives. Hopefully, this patient could be managed medically and would not have to come in for surgery, especially with the large foal inside her.

The next twelve hours would probably decide how the mare would do. She would have immediately been considered a surgical candidate if the pain meds and sedation had not affected her. When a horse is very painful, sedation and pain meds don't seem to work at all. If they were lucky, this girl would get to remain at home with no more problems.

Chapter 35

As they continued through their day, they stopped at several more farms. One was a dairy where they treated a cow with mastitis. Another farm had a horse with a hoof abscess. The girls got to castrate and deworm some calves at yet another farm. They stopped for lunch at a little country store. Sara ordered a bologna sandwich and chips. There was nothing like a thick piece of store bologna, some mayonnaise and fresh, white bread. Sara could feel the pounds adding on to her hips, but she didn't care. She would work those off this afternoon.

Dr. Rodriquez was particularly cheerful today. He asked the students plenty of questions on the things they saw and did, but they also got him to talk about Ames Plantation. He did not normally go to Ames with the students but a couple of years ago, Dr. Butler had been sick and Dr. Rodriquez had taken the students.

"It's a beautiful place - almost like stepping back in time. The bunkhouses where you stay are old guesthouses, and they're nice. No televisions or computers are in those houses. You walk back into history."

"No tvs? What do we do when we get through working? Just sit around and talk?" asked Hillary.

"No. They feed you and teach you about the plantation and how it used to be. You'll also have lectures at night and make plans about your next day, but you won't miss the tvs and the computers. They keep you so busy that when you go back to the bunkhouses all you want to do is go to bed. You're exhausted but in a good way, and believe me, you're belly is full. The food there is wonderful."

"That's what we've heard about the food, but really no tvs or computers? I'm not sure Ames is sounding that great." Sara said.

"You two will love it - guaranteed. They've got horses, cows, and pigs. You'll get all the practice you'll need and the horse barns are beautiful and cleaner than this little store."

"Really?"

"Yes, really. The hall of the barn is cobblestone and kept well. There are stained glass windows in parts of the barns, and the horses are in great shape. It doesn't even smell like a barn. You'll think you're in a museum."

"I'm ready to go." smiled Sara.

"It's an adventure, and one both of you need to go on. If I were either of you, I wouldn't pass it up. That's for sure."

They continued eating and talking and Sara and Hillary asked more questions about Ames. They more Dr. Rodriquez talked, the more they both wanted to go. Sara couldn't wait to get back to the clinic to find out the results of the draw, but she would have to. They had more work to do.

After lunch, they worked more calves, saw a couple more horses, and by four o'clock, headed back to the University. Sara knew the other students on her rotation had taken care of Quincy's two o'clock treatment, and no one had called, so she figured things had gone well.

When they got back to school, they said their good-byes to Dr. Rodriquez. This day was probably the last day they would get to ride with him. The rotation was coming to an end. Sara was sad about that. She had been so scared of him at first, and he had turned out to be one of the best professors she had the opportunity to work and ride with. She shook his hand and gave him a big smile. So did Hillary.

He smiled only for a minute and then turned and headed back to the office area to finish the day. He had many students before Hillary and Sara, and he would have many after. Sara and Hillary would remember Hector Rodriquez for years to come, as they would most of their professors. Hector Rodriquez would not remember them for long. There were too many of them, and the years rolled on.

Chapter 36

Hillary and Sara got back just in time to catch afternoon rounds. They would have to wait to see who was going to Ames until after rounds were finished. Several patients had been admitted for hospitalization.

Jessica had a horse with a large wound in its rump. Doug had a cow with pneumonia, and Josh had a goat with strange, neurological signs as well as a week old foal with diarrhea. The mare was also in the stall with her baby, and it was easy to see she was concerned.

Sara and Josh would be seeing a lot of each other in the halls at night now. A foal took a tremendous amount of care and could crash quickly. Both students would be putting in a lot of time for the rest of the rotation until their patients got better and went home.

Josh would probably need help with the treatments because the mare did not look like she was happy to have anyone touching her baby, and mares could be very dangerous animals when a baby was by their side. Sara would make sure she checked on Josh when she came back for her nightly treatments to Quincy.

The group finally made it to Quincy's stall. He was waiting for them, and he nickered as they approached.

"Treatment this afternoon went fine. His vitals are good, and he seems to be feeling good." Doug reported on Quincy since he had treated him while Sara was on ambulatory.

"Sounds good." Dr. Summers continued, "Okay, guys, we're done with rounds. Let's finish up the day, and I'll see y'all back tomorrow morning." Dr. Summers said, "and by the way, if you put your name in for Ames, they have the results of the drawing at reception."

Dr. Summers smiled a quirky, little smile and motioned for Hillary and Sara to go. She knew both girls had been drawn, but she wasn't going to tell them. She wanted the suspense to be drawn out just a little longer. Some things are better savored.

Hillary and Sara went straight to the reception desk, and there their names were on the list for Ames.

"Woohoo, girl!!!! We are going to Ames' plantation." Hillary grinned as she high-fived Sara's outstretched hand.

"This is going to be so much fun! I can hardly wait. We're going to be going back in time to an old southern plantation with lots of livestock and plenty of food!" Sara replied. "I'm so excited!"

"Me, too. I can't wait to get there. It'll be a good way to finish off this rotation, too. Get out of Knoxville, relax a little, work a lot, and eat till we pop."

"I'm going to need a little relaxation after Quincy. Maybe I can even sleep the whole drive down. That would be wonderful - some sleep." Sara said.

"You got that shot right." Hillary smiled at her friend.

Hillary knew Sara needed this trip as much or more than she did. Sara had been spending a lot of time treating Quincy and missing a lot of sleep. Sara was going on the fourth night in a row without more than three or four hours of sleep at a time. Even the night after she had emergency and was supposed to get a full nights rest, Jessica and Doug had to call for Quincy's treatment. Hillary could see the dark circles forming under Sara's eyes. Her friend was holding up well, but Hillary knew that Sara would soon need a break.

"Well, Sara, I don't know about you, but I think I'm going home to pack and start getting ready. You leaving or are you going to turn Quincy out for awhile?"

"I'm going to spend some time with the boy and let him graze some. I haven't seen him all day, and I know he wants outside. I'll start packing a little when I get home."

"Alright, well, I'll see you tomorrow, then." Hillary grinned. "Ames plantation, here we come!"

"See you tomorrow, Hillary." Sara grinned right back.

As Sara walked down the hall to Quincy's stall, pictures of old plantation homes and stately, picturesque barns danced in her mind. Ames would be so good for her. She was tired, and as she walked down that hall to her favorite patient, she started realizing how tired she was.

Quincy was better, and she was exhausted. She had pulled plenty of all-nighters studying during college, vet school, and now, down at the clinics, but she didn't think she had ever went without a good night's sleep for this long before. There was more to it than that, though, and Sara knew it. She wasn't just physically tired. She was emotionally drained.

Quincy had taken a lot from her. She had worried about him more than any other patient she had treated while in clinics, and she had fallen in love with this horse. She had been able to keep her distance with all of her other patients, but not him.

Sara was so happy he was doing better, and she wondered how veterinarians that had been practicing for years do what they do, but she knew. You just had to be strong - emotionally and physically, and that's all there was to it.

He was waiting for her as she approached his stall with lead rope in hand. He stood patiently as she capped off his iv line and snapped the lead rope to his halter. He put his head on her shoulder, and Sara stood there for a minute before she reached up and started gently rubbing his head and ears. Quincy did not move and girl and horse stood for a while breathing together.

After a few minutes, Sara turned and kissed Quincy on the nose and backed away.

"Okay, boy, let's go outside and get you some fresh, green grass."

Quincy obediently followed, but he wasn't pulling at the lead rope, and Sara noticed that he was walking slower.

"Whoa, boy. Hold on a minute. Let's go get my stethoscope."

Sara felt a small seed of terror rise in the pit of her stomach. He looked fine. Doug had said his vitals were good. He had eaten all his feed. Everything was fine, she was sure. He was just getting used to turn out again and not as excited about it as he was before. She had also been gone all day, and she was sure he had been looking for her. He was just tired.

Sara grabbed her stethoscope at the treatment station and listened to Quincy's lungs. Everything sounded fine, didn't it? Was she hearing a little more in those lungs than she did this morning? Was she being paranoid? She took his temp - all was normal. He was just tired.

"You sure you want to go out, Quincy? We don't have to. I'm tired, too. It's up to you."

Quincy turned his big head to the doors leading outside and took one step toward them then looked back at Sara.

"Okay, here we go."

They got outside to the grass and Quincy immediately started grazing. Sara could feel her tension start to ease. She watched his breathing carefully as he munched on the grass. It still wasn't completely normal but it was so much better than when he had come in. Everything was fine. He had just given her a little paranoid scare.

She sat down on the little hill and let her thoughts take her back to Ames. What did she need to pack? Confirm plans with Leanne for Jake. Call her parents and tell them about the trip. Would she need to take her laptop? Would she need to take any of her books or notes?

Sara planned as Quincy ate and before she knew it, they had been outside for a while. She looked at her watch. It was already 5:30. By the time she got Quincy back in, called Judy, and got home, it would be well after 6:00. She would have time for some supper, a little packing, and then before she knew it, she would have to be back here again.

"Come on, Quincy, let's go back in."

Quincy resisted for just a second, and Sara had to pull a little harder at his halter. His head came up from the grass, and he obediently followed Sara in. She got him set back up in his stall, rubbed his head, and turned to leave when she stopped in her tracks. Quincy had just coughed, and it wasn't a little hack. It was a deep down from the bottom of his toes cough.

Sara turned and looked at him. He looked back like nothing had just happened. She again got her stethoscope and thermometer.

Lungs sound okay and temperature is normal. She looked at him again. There was no noticeable change in his breathing or his attitude, and then she heard the voice. The voice from within her that she had kept quiet so well over the last two days now spoke.

"It is beginning again, Sara, and you know it."

The hair on the back of her neck stood up and that small seed of terror she had felt earlier now blossomed in the deepest pit of her stomach. She felt sick. She listened to his lungs yet again and took his temperature yet again. She turned and left the stall leaving Quincy with a quizzical look on his face. He wondered what was happening. His caretaker seemed very upset.

Sara returned with a small bucket of feed and some treats. She offered them to Quincy, and he was pleasantly surprised with his afternoon snack and treats. He ate them right up.

Sara gave him a pat on the head, some more hay, and closed the stall door behind her. She stood there watching him for another fifteen minutes. He quietly munched his hay and looked Sara's way. He loved her and was glad she was back. He had missed her today, but she was acting a little strange this afternoon. He was also hoping she didn't jump back in the stall to disturb him with that long rope thing she put to his chest and that annoying, little beeping thing she put in his rectum. He was getting pretty tired of that.

Quincy didn't cough anymore. He was eating and eating well. He was breathing well. He felt good. The voice was just a figment of her imagination. Everything was going so well with Quincy and with the Ames trip, Sara just figured her subconscious expected something to go wrong and so, it just threw a little wrench into the works.

She couldn't forget she was tired either. You just didn't think as rationally when you were tired. Sara ignored the fact that she was anything but tired now. That cough and the voice, even though it was wrong, had sent such a shot of adrenaline through Sara, she wasn't sure she would be able to sleep tonight, but she sure would try.

It was time to call Judy and then get home. She was ready to see Jake.

Chapter 37

"Hello."

"Hey, Mrs. Taylor, it's Sara. Just calling to check in."

"And how is Quincy doing, Sara?"

"He's doing good, Mrs. Taylor. I got to go to farms today, so I think he kinda' missed me, but he's eating well and breathing well. Hopefully, he'll get to go home soon."

"I'm sure he did miss you, Sara. He's getting used to you being there for him. Sounds like he's getting better and better, and the thought of bringing him home just makes me down right jittery with excitement. I can't wait to see him back in his own stall at home. Thank you so much, sweetheart."

"You're welcome, Mrs. Taylor, it has truly been my pleasure. Now, if you don't mind, I'm going to get off of here and get home. I'll call you first thing in the morning, and we'll go from there."

"Sure, Sara. I'll be waiting for your call."

As Sara hung up the phone, she hoped she sounded more confident to Judy than she felt right now. There was absolutely no reason to worry Judy. All Quincy's physical parameters were good and probably going to stay that way. He had done nothing but improve since he had gotten here. There was no reason to worry.

Sara went to her locker, got her stuff, and started to her truck. No reason to worry. No reason to worry. No reason to worry. She told herself again and again. As she pulled out onto the highway, she replayed that one cough in her head. She could talk and reason to herself all the way home, but one thing was for sure - she was worried.

As she drove through traffic, she tried to think of Ames, of Jake, of anything but Quincy, and about halfway home; she succeeded in thinking about something else. She, after all, would be back to check on him in less than two hours. Unless she decided to turn around, go back, and set with a horse that looked perfectly healthy all night, she had to make herself think about something else, and the thought of Ames was pleasant.

Sara planned which clothes she would take with her to Ames. They didn't have to wear the ugly, green coveralls at Ames, so she would need some pretty sturdy work clothes that she didn't mind getting dirty. She would take a jacket and toboggan in case it got cool, but there was no need to take any gloves. You couldn't do the kind of work they were going to do with a pair of heavy gloves.

Your hands just had to get cold, and you just had to put up with it. There was no way to have the dexterity in your hands you needed plus being cognizant of the feel of things with a pair of gloves on. She would need extra socks, an extra pair of boots, and the list continued. Before she knew it, she was at home.

Sara climbed the stairs, opened the door and greeted Jake. He was full of energy, so Sara extended their walk around the apartment complex. It was a beautiful, chilly spring evening, and Sara tried to relax. She needed to eat and call Leanne. She had about forty-five minutes until she had to head back to the clinic. She could accomplish the walk, supper, and the call in that time easy.

Sara knew she had to put things in perspective. Quincy was okay. She needed to enjoy her short time at home and calm down. She told herself this as she drug Jake back inside, started wolfing down a turkey sandwich with one hand and called Leanne with the other. She wanted to get back.

"Hello," Leanne answered.

"Hey, Leanne, it's me. Looks like I'm going to Ames." Sara told Leanne.

"That's great, Sara! Don't worry about Jake. You know I'll take care of him." Leanne assured Sara.

"I know. I just wanted to call and let you know for sure that I'll be gone."

"No problem. Y'all have a good time, okay, Sara?"

"Okay, Leanne. I'll talk to you later, and thanks."

"Sure, Sara. Have a good night."

"You, too."

Sara had finished her sandwich and was looking at her watch when she hung up with Leanne. She really did hope she was going to Ames, but she couldn't get Quincy out of her mind. She could hang out at her apartment for about fifteen more minutes before going back, but she knew it was pointless.

She could start packing some of her stuff, but she didn't want to. She wanted to go back and make sure Quincy was okay. She knew it was ridiculous. She hadn't been gone anytime, but she kept hearing that cough again and again - the cough that had come deep from within him. That cough that had seemed to rattle the stall door and start a tremor in Sara's world that she hoped didn't grow into an earthquake.

"Come on, Jake, let's take a ride." Sara commanded the pup.

The pup danced around the door as Sara hooked his leash to his collar. He was out the door and straining on his leash before Sara could get the door shut behind him.

"Jake, sit!" barked Sara.

Jake sat down immediately with the stern command and looked up at Sara with hurt eyes. He didn't understand why she was in such a mood, and he sure didn't understand why she was taking it out on him. He just wanted to go on a ride.

Sara felt guilty when Jake plopped down like he had been shot and looked up at her with those eyes. She shouldn't have issued the command so harshly, but she was tired, she was worried, and he was getting the brunt of her mood.

"I'm sorry, sweet baby. Momma is just tired and ill, and I shouldn't have taken it out on you. I'll do better, promise." Sara cooed to Jake.

She locked the door and swept him up in her arms. He planted puppy kisses around her nose and cheeks and let Sara hold him as she descended the steps of her apartment. As soon as they got in the parking lot, he jumped out of her arms. Sara was glad she had gotten him a retractable leash as she watched him run to the truck. When he got bigger, he might pull her arm out of its socket because of that retractable leash, but right now it was just good to see him have the freedom to jump and run.

Sara watched Jake as he headed to the truck. His little legs were growing and beginning to develop muscle. She watched the muscles move in perfect harmony as his little chest pumped with his effort of the run. His chest muscles were developing also, and he was starting to look like a lesson in anatomy class where they had to learn the names of all the muscles and how they worked together to propel an animal forward.

He stopped at the truck barely out of breath and waited for Sara to come and open the door. Sara stopped, too, when the comparison of Jake to Quincy came out of nowhere and struck her like a brick. Jake, early in life, had run and tugged her across the parking lot and there he stood - waiting, breathing completely normal now after exercise. His lungs, heart, muscles, and body were young. They had carried him easily where he needed to go with hardly any effort at all.

Quincy, on the other hand, had barely been able to walk into the exam room that first day. His lungs, heart, muscles, and body weren't young and they were diseased. Sara didn't know why, probably because of exhaustion, but the stark comparison of these two different animals hit her hard, and she felt a tear roll down her cheek.

Jake cocked his head, and both puppy ears stood straight up. He headed back to his mother in a cautioned and aware trot. Something was wrong, but he didn't know what.

Sara saw both ears stand up, and as Jake headed back to her, she begin to smile as another tear fell and then another.

"It's okay, buddy, momma's just gone crazy." She laughed and bent down to the pup.

Jake came to Sara and sensing her distress, stopped in front of her with a questioning stare.

"Come here, Jake, I'm okay. I just needed a minute." He came. Sara picked up the puppy and held him close as she walked to her truck. The few tears were drying up, and she felt the strength of his youth as she held him. She opened the truck door and climbed in with the pup in tow.

Jake, as usual, stayed in Sara's lap as she drove back to the clinic. She had to steady herself. She was going to go in and find a completely normal Quincy and all this blubbering was for nothing. She parked in the lot and left Jake in the truck. He wasn't particularly happy about the event, but the bone Sara threw him made it all better.

Chapter 38

Sara headed straight for Quincy's stall with her heart pounding in her chest. As she turned the corner, she called his name. She heard rustling from the stall, and then to her relief, Quincy popped his head out to watch Sara come to him.

"You're looking pretty good, ole' man. Been coughing any more? Let's take a look at you." Sara said to Quincy.

She examined him from head to toe and all seemed normal except one thing. His temperature was higher than it had been earlier this afternoon. It was still in the normal range for horses, but it was higher. Sara examined him again. All seemed well. She turned to Quincy.

"You feeling okay?"

Quincy just stared back.

"You look like you're breathing okay."

Quincy stared back.

"I've still got a couple of minutes until your treatment. I'm going to go check on Josh, and then I'm going to come down here again. Are you going to be okay?"

Quincy stared back at Sara. Sara stared at Quincy. Finally, Quincy turned to munch on his hay. If she wasn't going to treat him and just look at him, he could do that while he was eating.

That's a good sign, thought Sara. He's still eating like nothing's wrong, and that's probably because nothing is wrong. She stepped out of the stall and headed to the mare and foal Josh had taken in earlier that day. Quincy's temperature fluctuation worried her a little, but it wasn't that uncommon for their temp to go up and down as long as it stayed in the normal range. She would check it again when she treated him.

Sara had seen Josh's car when she had pulled into the parking lot, but she had wanted to check on Quincy before doing anything else. Quincy seemed to be fine, so she decided to see if

Josh was. Sara was pretty sure Josh had been at the clinics since morning. With the foal and the goat's treatment schedule, she doubted he had time to go home since afternoon rounds.

Stephanie and Josh were outside the foal and mare's stall talking when Sara came up and gave them a smile.

"How's it going?" she asked.

"It's going okay. The little fella' is holding on but momma sure doesn't like me messing with him. Me and Stephanie are about to give him his next treatment. I don't think either one of us would mind some help, if that's okay with you Sara." Josh said.

"No, problem, Josh. Stephanie, you on call tonight?" Sara asked.

"Yep, on call for large animal surgery. I was down in the surgery room cleaning up, and saw Josh wandering around looking like he was lost, so I thought he might need some help." Stephanie said.

"I'm not kidding y'all when I say this mare has had enough of us messing with her foal. I really didn't want to go in there by myself this time. Last time, she kept whirling around like she was figuring pretty hard on kicking my teeth out. I'm afraid this time she'll actually do it. I'm glad y'all are both here." Josh shyly grinned at the girls.

Josh had never been around horses and didn't plan on ever being around horses once he graduated, but he had a job to do tonight and the way it was looking, for the next several nights. He would do his job, and he would do his job well but any help he might get from anybody around was appreciated.

"Okay, y'all ready?" Asked Josh.

"You got all your stuff? Last thing we need if she's going to be hard to deal with is us getting in there and you not having all your stuff together." Stephanie asked Josh.

He patted the pockets on his overalls, shook his head, and said, "Got it all."

"Alright, here we go." said Stephanie.

She motioned for Sara to open the stall door, and as she did, the mare who had been standing in the corner with her foal behind her, looked Sara's way and backed her ears so far back on her head, it was hard to tell she had ears.

"You better be quick guys. She looks really unhappy." Sara said.

Sara had barely gotten the words out and Stephanie had barely gotten into the stall when the mare charged. One thousand and four hundred pounds of pure muscle rushed at the students with her ears back and her teeth bared. The mare was biting at the air so hard, her teeth made a popping sound that resembled a rifle going off inside the stall. The noise was both deafening and chilling at the same time.

Sara held the door open, and Stephanie rushed back through. They all looked at each other.

"Uh-oh." Sara said with her eyes wide and her heart racing.

"I told you she was getting tired of me. What are we going to do now?" Josh asked.

And then Sara heard a man with a Spanish accent say, "What's going on down there? Did I hear some kind of gun go off?"

It was Dr. Rodriquez. Stephanie, Sara, and Josh all sighed a sigh of relief.

"No, sir. This mare wants to kill us with her teeth or her feet. She's not caring which one really." Josh answered him.

A smile spread across Dr. Rodriquez's mouth, and he shook his head. "Are y'all trying to have some fun without me?"

"No, sir. In fact, I was just coming to get you. I thought you'd probably still be here." Stephanie said. "The mare doing okay?"

"Yes, yes, she's doing fine. Will is recovering her. I think her baby will be fine, too, but we'll just have to see. Sara and I saw her this morning actually. You remember her, Sara?" He asked.

"Huh?" Sara had no idea what they were talking about.

"The mare we saw with colic on ambulatory this morning had to come in for surgery tonight. She got better and then got worse again, so the owners brought her in. That's why Will, Stephanie, and me are here. We are all on surgery call, and it looks like that is a very good thing for you, Josh, huh?"

"Yes, sir, a very good thing."

"Okay, let's see what we can do with this girl. Let me have a look." Stephanie and the students backed out of the way and gave Dr. Rodriquez some room.

First, he started talking to the mare in a low, Spanish whisper. She looked like she was calming down. Then, he slowly opened the stall door, still talking to her. She stood looking at him for only a minute, and then she charged him, too. Dr. Rodriquez could really move when he had to.

"Whew, this girl is mad, isn't she? Josh what have you been doing to her? Beating her baby?" Dr. Rodriquez teased Josh.

"Nope, she just gets a little bit meaner every time I touch the baby and now I think she may be fed up." Josh replied.

"I think you're right." Dr. Rodriquez agreed. "Stephanie, go get me some drugs. Sara, go get me a twitch, and Josh go get me a lasso. I'm going to get a ladder. Meet you all back here in about five minutes."

Chapter 39

They all scattered to get supplies and met back at the stall. Dr. Rodriquez was setting up the ladder in the adjacent stall that was empty. He climbed to the top of the ladder and looked down into the mare and foal's stall. The three wondered what he was going to do next.

"Okay, Josh, hand me the lasso."

Josh handed him the lasso. The mare was looking at Dr. Rodriquez intently and so were the students and Stephanie. He began again talking to the mare in a low, Spanish whisper while working the lasso closer and closer to the mare's head. He did not raise the lasso high in the air and swing it several times and then throw it like you see in rodeos. He just slow pitched it over the mare's head. She didn't hear it coming but she sure felt it when it landed. She quickly backed up which tightened the lasso around her neck. Dr. Rodriquez gave her some slack, and she quit backing up.

"Okay, I'm going to work the end of the rope over to the stall door, and we'll see what to do from there." He climbed down from the ladder and kept hold of the other end as he stepped it to the stall door. The man was tall with a long reach and the stalls weren't very high. It would have been impossible for someone shorter to pull off.

"Now, I want you all to stay out of the stall, and see what I can do with her. Sometimes, once they know you've got them, it will calm them down. Let's see how this goes."

The mare was watching them closely as Dr. Rodriquez opened the stall door a crack and tightened up on the rope all the while talking to the mare in a low whisper. The mare did not charge but stubbornly inched forward as he pulled on the rope. Stephanie, Sara, nor Josh moved a muscle. They just watched.

Once he got the mare close enough to reach out and touch her, Dr. Rodriquez slowly started rubbing the mare on the head. She was not happy, but she let him, and before anyone knew it, he had turned the loop around her neck into a halter. He was now beside the mare and held her snuggly.

"Okay, Sara, hand me the twitch - SLOWLY."

Sara inched the twitch through the door. He was able to get the twitch around the mare's ear. She wasn't moving but she was breathing very hard and everyone knew there was a chance for her to explode at any time.

"Stephanie, step in with the drugs and give them."

Stephanie cautiously moved into the stall and had given the drugs intravenously before anyone could hardly see her hand move. Thirty seconds later, they could all see the mare start calming down.

After a minute, Dr. Rodriquez removed the twitch and asked for a halter. He skillfully placed the halter with lead rope on the mare and removed the lasso.

"Okay, guys, do what you need to do with the baby. I'll keep this girl occupied."

Stephanie and Josh moved into the stall like covert operatives. They had the foal treated in no time and were back outside the stall. Dr. Rodriquez still had the mare but she was beyond caring at this point. The drugs were doing their job.

Dr. Rodriquez tied the mare to one of the bars in the stall near the food and water. He did not leave her enough slack to be able to step on the rope or get tangled in it, but he did leave her enough slack to be able to eat and drink and check on her baby. He stepped out of the stall.

"That should help you some with her tonight, Josh. The sedation won't last until the next treatment, and we can't keep her knocked out for days on end. You need to make sure someone is here with you when you treat them but keeping her tied should help you get a hold of her easily enough. Hopefully, when she sees she can't do anything to you and that her baby is getting better, she will calm down. Most of these mares get better in just a couple of days, but if she doesn't, you're in for a lot of fun." Dr. Rodriquez said with a smile.

"Nothing to get the blood pumping like a mare wanting to kill you. What a night!" Dr. Rodriquez laughed out loud. "Anybody else need help while I'm here?"

Sara was not over the excitement with the mare and foal. Her heart was still racing, so she nearly missed his offer for help - nearly.

"Since you're here, and if you don't mind, could you look at this horse I've been treating?" Sara asked.

Dr. Rodriquez cocked his head and smiled. "Sure, Sara, I'll look at your horse, but let's all take a breath first."

"Amen." Josh piped in.

So, they stood there - Josh, Stephanie, Sara, and Dr. Rodriquez, and they watched the little foal. The mare was still pretty out of it, but she still noticed her sick baby waddling up beside her. She nickered at him, and he nickered back. He went to his mother's udder and began to nurse. The mare closed her eyes and began to relax even more as her baby who was not acting normal now did something completely normal.

The rhythmic sound of the foal nursing his mother, the most natural sound in the world, seemed to relax them all. They watched him as he bumped his mother's udder with his nose signaling his desire for more milk. They watched him as he finished, gave a little smack, and yawned. The little man was tired after an eventful day, and it was time for a nap.

Dr. Rodriquez sighed and nodded to Sara, "Let's go."

"Hey, Doc, thanks a lot. I don't know what I would have done if you hadn't been here." Josh called after him.

"You would have figured it out Josh." Dr. Rodriquez called back to Josh as he and Sara headed to Quincy's stall.

Sara realized again that in just a couple of months, they wouldn't have Dr. Rodriquez to call for back up. In certain situations, they might have no one to call. They would have to figure it out, but right now, she did have Dr. Rodriquez, and she was going to use him.

Chapter 40

They stood at Quincy's stall, and Sara filled Dr. Rodriquez in on Quincy's history, treatments, and condition.

"I can tell he's much better, and he's been getting much better all along, but this afternoon, I heard him cough, and it wasn't just a weak, little hack. It was a pretty bad cough, and now tonight, his temp is up a little. I'm pretty sure I'm worried about nothing, but it would be nice to get another opinion." Sara told Dr. Rodriquez.

"Okay, let's have a look." Dr. Rodriquez did a complete exam of Quincy, taking his time, which Sara appreciated. She knew it was late, and he probably had other things to do tonight, but he was making time for a student.

"He sounds okay, Sara. He's got some stuff in his lungs, but that's to be expected with what he's been through. His temp is the same as it was earlier, so it's not rising. He seems okay to me. I would just treat him and keep a close eye on him like you've been doing."

"Thanks, Dr. Rodriquez, that makes me feel a lot better."

"You're welcome, Sara, my pleasure. I hope I've helped."

"You have." Dr. Rodriquez was turning to leave the stall. "I'll be able to sleep tonight."

He grinned and turned back to Sara. "I want you to sleep tonight, Sara, but I'm going to let you in on a little secret, okay?"

"Okay."

"You know that mare we saw this morning and then had to do surgery on tonight?"

"Yes, sir."

"When we left the farm this morning, I had no worries that I would be doing surgery on that mare tonight. She responded beautifully to treatment, felt great when we left, gut sounds better, and was normal. I'm usually right, but sometimes they trick you. They are supposed to do what the books say they are supposed to do, but you know what, Sara?"

"Hmmm?"

"They don't all read the book. Where would be the challenge if they did, huh? Keep an eye on your boy."

"Yes, sir."

"See ya later, Sara."

"See ya', Dr. Rodriquez."

He walked off down the hall, and Sara could hear his boots echoing against the concrete floors. So, sometimes, no matter how smart we are or think we are, sometimes no matter how hard we work, no matter how hard we try, and no matter how long we do this job, thought Sara, we still get surprises or as Dr. Rodriquez put it - challenges. Great.

"Need to be reading the book, Quincy, cause the book says you're getting better." Sara smiled at her boy. "Okay, let's get this treatment over. We're a little late because of crazy, momma mare."

Sara treated Quincy, gave him more hay, and a couple of treats. She spent some time stroking his neck and rubbing him under the chin. Dr. Rodriquez had definitely eased Sara's mind, and she had not heard Quincy cough a single time since she had been there. It was time to get out of here and try to grab a couple hours of sleep before the next treatment.

Sara checked on Josh before she left. Everything seemed fine. The mare was less sedated, but seemed at ease with the situation. Her sick baby was sleeping heavily curled up in the hay beside his mother. Josh was also going to leave and try to get something to eat and maybe a little sleep before coming back. He was scheduled to treat the foal again at one a.m., and Will had assured him he would be around monitoring the mare that had surgery earlier.

Josh and Sara walked together out to their vehicles talking about the close call with the mare and how easily one could get hurt working with these animals. The well known saying for those that worked with large animals was "it's not when are you going to get hurt, it's how bad are you going to get hurt" because it goes without saying, you will get hurt.

"Why do you want to do it, Sara? Why not stick to just dogs and cats when you get out of here?" Josh asked Sara when they had both arrived at their vehicles.

"I've always wanted to do it, Josh. Don't know exactly why. I don't know if it's because I grew up with them, or because I know my way around them. Now don't get me wrong, I want to work on dogs and cats, too, but there is just something about a farm, the fields, the smell, and the animals. I don't know. I just know I do." Sara told Josh.

"Well, if me and Will get killed tonight with that mare, I want you to remember me, okay?" Josh asked with a smile.

"I'll remember you Josh, and don't worry, Will knows his way around a horse."

"Thank God." Josh replied. "See you tomorrow, Sara."

"See you, Josh."

Jake was impatiently waiting for Sara to get in the truck. There were paw prints and nose prints all over the driver's side windows. The bone had been gone for some time.

"Scoot over, buddy, momma's coming in."

Jake obediently went to the passenger's seat, and as soon as Sara was buckled in, he jumped in his place in her lap. They drove home in silence. She let Jake do his duty outside, and then carried him into the apartment. Sara changed into her pajamas, slid in between the sheets, set the alarm for one a.m. and quickly went to sleep. It was 9:30 p.m.

Chapter 41

Sara was on the riverbank again, and she knew it was a dream.

"Wake up!! Wake up!!! Wake up!!!!" She yelled to herself. It wasn't working.

Sara began to pinch herself on the riverbank. That wasn't working either. I don't want to dream this dream again. I definitely do not want to dream this dream again she told herself, but it was useless. She was still on the riverbank.

When her mind realized it was not getting out of this dream, Sara started noticing the dream had changed. It was no longer raining, and it didn't look like it was going to. The rain had passed. The ground around her was still muddy and the river was still trying to bulge over the banks, but the roaring of the clouds and the river had ceased.

A fog had settled around the river and the bank, but Sara could still see the band of horses on the other side. The leader was staring right at Sara, but he wasn't screaming at her, he was staring calmly.

Sara felt a chill run down her back as she stared back. The leader was calm, too calm, and all the other horses were behind him in a semi-circle. They were calm, too. Sara had no idea how this dream was going to go, but she could feel the ominous mood surrounding her, and she didn't like it.

They stood there, Sara and the horses, staring at each other for what seemed like an eternity. The sky was still overcast, and the rain had brought a chill to the air. The fog was getting thicker, but Sara could still see their shadows as they stood. She could hear as one or two pawed the ground and as another whinnied. Their breath made puffs of smoke within the fog. They were waiting on something.

Then, Sara heard a horse call out from beyond the group, far past the bank, away on a hill. She couldn't see the horse. It was too far away, and the fog was too thick. The whole group turned from Sara to the horse on the hill. Sara could hear him approaching, first as his hoofs hesitantly descended the hill, and then as he began to gallop toward the group. The group called to him, he called back. He sounded so familiar to Sara, but she couldn't place the horse. She had heard so many in her life.

As Sara was listening intently, she saw movement from the fog. The leader had turned back to her while the rest of the group looked toward the approaching horse. The fog cleared around him and the leader stepped forward. He looked at Sara and then from deep in his chest came a challenging roar that made Sara shake with terror. She felt her heart sink into her stomach, and her breath stopped. She became cold, and afraid, and sad all in one moment, and she began to cry from the terror and sadness, and she didn't know why. A strange, beeping noise began infiltrating her dream. Sara awoke to her one a.m. alarm.

Chapter 42

Jake watched Sara as she changed clothes and got ready to go back to the clinic. He looked pretty satisfied lying on the pillow on the bed. She gave him a questioning glance, stepped outside the room, and listened to see if he was going to try and follow. He never moved. The little pup was tired, and Sara decided to let him rest.

The night air had gotten colder, and Sara was glad she had grabbed her jacket as she walked out to the truck. Sara looked up at the full moon and the stars. They were gorgeous, but tonight, they only made her feel small and lonely. No other lights were on around the apartment, and Sara felt as if she were alone in a great, big world. She knew that wasn't true, but the dream had left her with a real sense of loneliness and melancholy. She climbed in her truck and turned the ignition.

As she drove to the clinic for what seemed like the thousandth time in three days, she was well aware that she was one of the very few people that were out this time of night, and she also knew that when she graduated, this trend would continue. Veterinarians worked long hours and mixed animal practitioners worked really long hours.

The veterinarians at home had come in oftentimes with red, swollen eyes and a huge mug of coffee while walking straight to the coffee maker to make more. She had heard stories about delivering calves by the moonlight, treating cut horses by flashlight, and doing C-sections on dogs at two and three o'clock in the morning. She had seen them some nights at the clinic as she drove by on her way to friends homes or out to eat or going to the movies. Their trucks would be parked in front and the lights would be on out back. Sometimes she would stop to see what was going on, and sometimes she would drive on by.

Most of the time when she stopped, they would be stocking their trucks to go on a farm call or sitting in the horse room watching a horse on iv fluids or in pain or watching for a foal to be born. It didn't matter the time; it didn't matter the weather; it didn't matter if they were missing an anniversary or a wedding, a birthday or a ball game, they came and they helped and they did what needed to be done. Sara respected them tremendously, and in a few short months, she was going to be one of them.

    Tonight, however, she didn't feel like one of them. She felt lonely and worried and a little afraid of what she might find when she went back to the clinic to check on Quincy, but she was on her way there. She was going to help, she was going to do what needed to be done, and she was going to keep on doing what needed to be done.

Chapter 43

Quincy was standing in the center of the stall. His breathing appeared to be coming with a fraction of more effort. Tiny beads of sweat slowly ran down his neck and back. He did not walk to Sara and meet her when she opened the stall door.

She walked up to him with stethoscope and thermometer in hand and let out a long, tired sigh. He rested his head on her shoulder as she reached up to stroke his damp neck. He felt hot to her touch, and her heart sank.

"Okay, Quincy, let me see what's going on."

Sara examined him. She listened to his lungs and in just a few hours, she could hear more crackles than she had before. His temperature had shot up two degrees and was no longer in the normal range. She didn't care if it was two o'clock in the morning; she was going to call Dr. Summers.

"You hold on, fella', this is just a little bump in the road. I'm going to call Dr. Summers, and we're going to make you feel better." Her voice was shaky and she felt a tear run down her cheek. Quincy looked at her with a knowing look in his eyes.

She made it to the phone in the hall in no time. Everyone's number was there. She had left her cell phone in the truck. She dialed her number. A sleepy Dr. Summers answered with "Hello."

"Dr. Summers, it's Sara. Quincy has more crackles in his lungs and his temperature is up. He was coughing at five, but he checked out okay. At eight, his exam was normal with no coughing. Now, he is sweating just a little, and I can tell he's breathing with more effort. What do I need to do?"

"Sara, if it weren't two in the morning, I would ask you that, but since it is two in the morning, I'm going to tell you what you already know to do." Replied Dr. Summers.

Sara and Dr. Summers talked for about twenty minutes, and Dr. Summers told Sara exactly what medications to give Quincy and how much. She told her to increase his iv fluid rate, stay with him for about an hour to make sure his fever started coming down and call her if he got worse.

"Meet me at seven in the morning, Sara. I'll be in early to check him, and we'll go from there." Dr. Summers paused, "Sara, you okay?"

Sara knew Dr. Summers was on her side. Sometimes, not often, but sometimes it felt with the professors, clinicians, residents, and interns that it was students against them. Tonight, the concern and sincerity in Dr. Summers voice caught Sara off guard, and she heard her voice crack as she replied, "Yes, ma'am, I'm fine."

There was another pause as Julia Summers thought about whether she needed to come in and help this student with this horse. Julia had no doubt that Sara was completely competent, and she would do exactly what she told her to do. Julia knew Sara was having a hard time with this turn of events and especially since it was Quincy, but Julia also knew that Sara needed to go this alone. She didn't need a babysitter anymore, and so, Julia closed the conversation with, "I'll see you in the morning, Sara."

"Yes, ma'am." Sara hung up the phone and walked to the treatment station. Her hands were shaking as she took the medications off the shelf and drew them up in the syringe. She didn't have to have a pharmacy request for these medications. These were the ones that were stocked in every treatment station for emergencies. These were medications that you could easily get to when you didn't have time to walk to the pharmacy if it were open or that you needed when the pharmacy was closed, like two o'clock in the morning. These medications meant you had an unscheduled problem on your hands, and most of the time, a serious problem.

She walked back to Quincy's stall feeling like she was in an alternate universe. Not five hours before, she had walked out of this place a little worried, but all in all, feeling fine - feeling better. Now, she felt as if a fifty-pound weight was sitting on her chest and someone had hollowed out her insides. She was in an alternate universe where the animals and those hateful organisms that make them sick, don't read the book, and she didn't like this universe - not at all.

Quincy was right where she had left him. He had not taken one step. She smiled a sad smile as she entered the stall and began to give him medications as she cooed to him in her softest voice.

"I know you feel kinda' funny right now, fella', but we're going to make you feel better. I'm going to give you some stuff to get that temperature down a little and some stuff to soothe you. I'm going to stay right here with you, and you're gonna' do fine, just fine. You're a big, strong boy. This is just a little set back. Me and you both know it was probably going too easy. This is just a little bump in the road. I believe in you. We're going to be fine."

Sara stayed with him - a girl and a horse in the middle of the night at a veterinary referral center. She stroked his neck for a long time, then she went and got a brush and started going over his body in smooth, long strokes. Her daddy had taught her how to brush a horse, and she had done it so many times, it was almost like breathing to her. She let herself get lost in the rhythmic strokes and watched with satisfaction as the drugs took hold, and Quincy's breathing got easier and the small droplets of sweat dried up.

She heard Josh and Will come in to treat the mare in the hospital stalls two rows back. She heard them talking low to the mare and didn't hear a lot of commotion, so she knew everything went fine. She never let them know she was there. She didn't want to see anyone, and she didn't want to talk to anyone. She just wanted to stay with Quincy.

After she had finished brushing him, she combed out his mane and tail. He would have looked pretty good if not for the fact that he had no fat left on his body. His ribs could easily be seen through his coat, and Sara had taken special care to brush softly around these bones. His hipbones also stood starkly out against his rump even though he had gained weight in the few short days he had been there, it was obvious to anyone that knew anything about a horse that Quincy had been through it.

Sara took a deep breath and exhaled slowly through her mouth. She stepped back from Quincy and looked at her watch. It had been an hour since she had given the meds. She could tell from how Quincy was acting that his temperature would be back down, but she checked it anyway. She was right.

He looked better, and he looked comfortable, and this gave Sara some hope for him. It wasn't uncommon in animals or people to have a backset but that didn't mean it was time to give up. As far as Sara was concerned with this horse, it would take a lot more than this to give up. Dr. Summers would meet her in the morning, and they would fix this. They would run the tests they needed to run and find out exactly what was going on. They would then treat him, and he would turn around. He still wanted to live, and his heart was big. He wasn't giving up and neither was she.

"Okay, Quincy. You're looking better. I'm going home because I am exhausted, and I don't think me being here is going to do you or me any good. You going to be okay while I'm gone?"

Quincy looked at Sara, and she thought she saw a flicker of a question in his eyes, but then it was strong Quincy looking back at her again.

"I'll see you in the morning, fella'."

Sara left the clinic and went home.

Chapter 44

The alarm woke her up at 6:00 a.m. She had gotten home at three and quickly fallen asleep. Sara was amazed she had been able to sleep at all, but she had. Exhaustion was funny that way. No matter how worried she was about Quincy, her body demanded that sleep trump everything else. Sara had no problem sleeping instead of eating, sleeping instead of watching television, sleeping instead of picking up her apartment, sleeping instead of packing for Ames.

Ames. What was she going to do about Ames? They were supposed to leave in the morning. She would just have to talk to Dr. Butler about it and see what he thought. She wasn't going to leave Quincy if he wasn't doing better, and she wasn't sure she was going to leave Quincy even if he was.

She had planned on Quincy going home today or tomorrow with Judy and now Sara seriously doubted if that was going to happen. If he were well enough to go home with Judy, Sara would have no worries.

Judy. What was she going to say to Judy? The thought of talking to Judy and telling her that Quincy was worse was about as bad as Quincy being worse. How that woman loved this horse, and she, Sara, was going to have to tell her, but she didn't know what to tell her yet. He might be better this morning, but he might not be. Sara would just have to see how Quincy was, tell Judy the truth, and go from there.

As she was thinking about Ames and Judy, Sara felt a warm, little tongue darting in and out of her ear. Someone else was up, too.

"Okay, Jake, let me get on my jacket, and we'll go outside. You can't walk for long, though, cause I got to get to the clinic." Jake jumped off the bed easily. Besides both ears standing now, his legs had grown. He was getting bigger. In just four days, the pup had grown.

As soon as Jake got to the grass, he started taking care of business. It didn't take long until Jake was done with business and started exploring around the landscaping. Spring was definitely coming to Knoxville, even if the morning air did have a bite. There were flowers popping up everywhere, and Jake needed to explore each new blossom. Sara smiled and took a deep breath of the spring air to calm herself, to remind her of the fields of flowers at home.

Then she remembered. The last time she had breathed deep to calm herself and be reminded of home was the morning she had met Quincy, and since that time, he had inserted himself firmly in her life. He had taken most of her time, and he was worth it. She needed to get back to the clinic, and check on her boy.

"C'mon, Jake. It's time to go back in. Sorry." Sara said apologetically to Jake.

He pulled against the leash, but when Sara firmly tugged him, he came obediently.

"I know you're tired of me never being here and when I am here, sleeping, but this is going to be over pretty soon, buddy. I'll be off the rotation in a couple more days, and I'll get to spend more time with you."

Sara would be off the rotation in a couple of more days whether she went to Ames or not or whether Quincy got better or not. That was just one more thing to worry about. What if Quincy wasn't better when it was time for her next rotation? Well, that was one thing she was not going to worry about now. She would worry about that later. Now, it was time to get ready for work.

Sara and Jake returned to the apartment. She quickly showered, left off the make-up, and got dressed. At this point, make-up was the last thing she was worried about. Sara looked at her face in the mirror and smiled. She looked awful, but she had seen all her classmates look the same way. They had gotten used to seeing each other at their best and at their worst.

As she drove to the clinic, Sara thought about how they had all looked the first year in vet school. She remembered that for at least the first couple of weeks, they dressed up in nice pants or skirts. Most of the women had their make-up on and their hair done. Most of the men had on khakis and dress shirts.

Then, the first big test came. Some came in looking disheveled, but not too bad. Then, the second big test came. There were some ponytails and jeans, some tennis shoes and sandals, and so it went. By the time they had all gotten to third year, everyone had seen each other without make-up, disheveled, unshaved, and many times, manure and or urine covered.

By the time they got to clinics, nobody cared what they looked like. They were all just tired. Sara, Hillary, Leanne, and Seth had laughed and laughed when they had gotten their senor pictures and compared them to their incoming first year identification badges.

"It's like the pictures of the presidents you see after their four-year terms. Man, have we aged!!! We don't even look like the same people." Seth had roared.

"We look like kids on our i.d. badges and old people in our senior pictures. It would be like aging ten years in four." Sara had agreed.

"Look at the grey in my hair!!! Is my hair really that grey?" Leanne had seriously asked.

"Nothing a bottle can't cure, my dear." Hillary had laughed and replied.

They had aged, and there was no denying that, and as Sara pulled into the parking lot, she knew exactly why. The stress had been tremendous. The stress of failing had been like a dark, deep cloud surrounding them all the first three years.

Make one F in vet school, and you're gone. Make one D, and you better not make another or guess what? You're gone. You had to maintain grades, and you had to do the work. Sara remembered that one of her tests in one of her classes had covered six hundred and seventy pages of notes, and that wasn't even a mid-term or a final, but as she walked to the clinic to see what was waiting for her, she almost wished for that type of stress again. She had some control over the grades that she made her first three years. She just had to study and study hard.

She had a weary, resounding suspicion that sometimes, in cases like Quincy, she had no control whatsoever, and no matter how hard she worked, it may not matter. Sometimes, it was all up to the great practitioner in the sky, and that was just how it was.

She rounded the corner and heard a deep cough. She didn't have to wonder which stall it was coming from. She called to him and his head did not pop out the stall door. She stood at his stall and took it all in.

Chapter 45

He was sweating this morning and not small drops just on his neck and back. The sweat wasn't rolling off of him and puddling on the floor, but he was sweating. His breathing was raspy, and it was an effort for him to inhale and exhale. He was still better than when he had come to them, but there was no denying that he was getting worse.

Sara stepped into his stall and patted her friend on top of his head. He looked at her with imploring eyes.

"Okay, fella', let's get to work."

His temperature was up again this morning and his lungs sounded worse. He was half-heartedly munching on some hay, and he didn't want his grain at all. He had literally eaten like a horse yesterday morning. The meds Sara gave him should have kept his temperature down for at least six to seven hours. It had barely been four. They needed a new plan.

"Good morning, Sara, how we doin'?" Sara heard Dr. Summers walk into the stall.

"Not too good."

"Move over and let me see."

Dr. Summers listened to Quincy's chest for what seemed to be hours to Sara. She checked him over from head to toe as Sara patiently waited.

"What do we need to do for him now, Sara?" she asked.

"I think we need to do another x-ray, more bloodwork, and possibly a transtracheal wash to find out exactly what kind of bug we have doing this and what kind of antibiotic is going to kill it."

"Good. Do you think the COPD is getting worse, or do you think the infection is getting worse?"

"With the temperature, I would go with the infection even though he may be breathing with such effort that it's raising his temperature, but I don't really believe that. I think the bloodwork, x-rays, and wash results will help us with that."

"You're right. Go ahead and get the bloodwork and x-rays set up. I'll get the wash set up, and I'm calling Dr. Sneed down to have a look at him. This morning, go ahead with his regular treatments and add another fever reducer. Hold off on any sedatives, though, because I think we will get his procedures underway quickly, and we will need to sedate him for those. You need to call his owner after treatments, and we'll keep each other posted. If you don't make it to morning rounds, I'll know you're busy, so let's get going."

"You got it."

Sara pulled the blood, treated Quincy, gave a heads up to radiology and in no time, found herself at the phone dialing Judy's number.

"Hello." answered Judy.

"Mrs. Taylor, it's Sara."

"Well, hello, Sara, you're calling kinda' early this morning. You ready for me to come get my boy and want me there before closing time?" Asked Judy.

Sara could hear the excitement in Judy's voice. She closed her eyes, took a deep breath and said, "No, ma'am. He started getting a little worse late last night, and this morning, he's quite a bit worse. We caught it early last night, though, and are treating him aggressively. We are going to do some more tests today and go from there. I still think he's going to be fine. We're just having a little bump in the road, that's all."

There was silence on the line, and then she heard Judy softly sobbing.

"Sara," Judy said in a broken voice, "I'm going to put my husband on the phone for a minute. I can't talk right now. You tell him what you told me."

"Yes, ma'am." Sara felt like she was going to die.

"Hello, this is Mr. Taylor."

"Hello, Mr. Taylor. This is Sara, and I've been taking care of Quincy. He's worse today, and we would like to do more tests to find out exactly what we're dealing with and go from there. Is that okay with y'all?"

"Yes, Sara. Whatever it takes. Do you still think he's going to be okay?" he asked.

"He's still a lot better than when he came in Mr. Taylor. I think we are probably just having some minor problems, but we need to look into it further." Sara replied.

"Okay, Sara. Hold on. Judy can talk now, and she wants to talk to you for just a minute. That okay?"

"Sure, Mr. Taylor."

Sara held her breath as she heard Judy get back on the phone.

"Sara, do you remember what I asked you to do for me?"

"Yes, ma'am. You told me to take care of your boy."

"I sure did, Sara, and I know you have done that. Do you remember what else I asked you to do?"

Sara felt a tear slide down her cheek, but her voice was still strong as she answered Judy.

"Yes, ma'am. You said for me to make sure your boy didn't suffer."

"So, Sara, I ask you now. Is he suffering?"

"He's sick, Mrs. Judy, but he is still nibbling hay, and he is still pretty strong. I wouldn't give up on him yet."

"Okay, Sara. You let me know about those tests today, and you keep me informed, understand."

"Yes, Mrs. Judy, you know I will."

"I do, Sara. I think you love him too, don't you?"

Another tear slid down Sara's cheek.

"Yes, ma'am. I do."

"I'll talk to you later."

"Okay, Mrs. Taylor."

Sara hung up and felt tears welling up fast in her eyes. She had just delivered the news that had rocked Judy Taylor's world, and it was such hard news to deliver. One thing Sara knew for sure - she would do right by Quincy, and she would do right by Judy Taylor, and that meant doing everything she could do for Quincy.

Sara checked her watch. She had indeed missed morning rounds. She needed to check with Dr. Summers about incoming patients. She needed to find her, but first, she was going to check on Quincy one more time.

Sara went down to his stall, and he was gone. They had probably already taken him to radiology or for the wash. His iv line was hanging from the bag twisting slowly with the light breeze that blew through his stall. Sara could see his hoof prints leading from the stall, and it seemed so strange to be standing at the door of his stall and him not in it. A sense of loneliness descended on Sara like a blanket.

It had only been four days, but it seemed now like four months. She had always been treating Quincy, it seemed to Sara. She had always been coming back for or just staying in the clinics to do the eight o'clock treatments and always been waking up to do the two a.m. treatments. She had spent hours in this stall, around this stall, and outside with this horse, and now he wasn't there. The stall seemed so empty.

Once again, Sara felt the tears start to come, and she choked them back and down. He was going to be fine. She was working on no sleep, not much food, and adrenaline. Everything seemed worse than it really was. She needed to get herself together and find Dr. Summers. Dr. Summers would know exactly where Quincy was and how Sara needed to go about her day.

Chapter 46

Julia Summers was in the break room waiting for Sara to find her. She had called Dr. Sneed several times and had yet to get an answer. He was the main clinician on this horse, and he needed to take a look at him. Julia doubted if he had even made it to work yet. She was leaving a message on his phone as Sara walked into the door.

"They have him in radiology, Sara, and they have him pretty sedated. He didn't want to leave with Seth, who is probably getting a complex with this horse by now, but they gave him some good stuff, and they got him to go. The wash is scheduled right after radiology. I wish you could be there for that, but the surgery rotation will take care of that procedure.

After they get done with him there, he should be back in his stall, and I put a STAT request on his bloodwork. When we get all those results in, I'll let you know, and we'll go from there.

In the meantime, we have patients to see, if you've called Mrs. Taylor."

"I've called her, and she says do what we need to do."

"Good, now, let's get started with your day."

"Yes, ma'am."

Sara went to the reception area and called the next client. It was a cow that was running a high temperature and not eating. The cow's nose and gums were white with anemia. Sara had seen this problem several times at home, quickly diagnosed the problem, got Dr. Summer's approval, and administered treatment. Then, she went to the next patient.

The next patient was a llama, which Sara knew nothing about. She did the best she could with the physical exam, listened to the client, and came up with a list of differentials. She went through them with Dr. Summers, they did more test, diagnosed the problem, and treated the llama. Then, she went to the next patient.

And so the morning went on. Sara saw several patients. She did her exams, she came up with her diagnoses and treatments, and she did her job. Sara was sure the clients could not tell part of her mind was elsewhere. She listened when she was supposed to be listening, nodded when she was supposed to nod, and instructed the clients on the care of their animals. All the while, a large part of her attention and her mind was on Quincy, but Sara was able to cover her thoughts well. Vet school taught you how to do that.

Finally, a break in the schedule allowed Sara to have lunch and check on Quincy. Sara didn't care about eating. She just wanted to see how Quincy was doing.

He looked worse. He was still sedated from the procedures, but he looked worse. He was holding his head down and his bottom lip hung down lower than it should. He was still sweating, partly from his condition and partly from the sedation. He did not acknowledge Sara as she entered the stall, and maybe this scared her the most. Quincy seemed in another world. She quickly did her exam. His temperature was going up, and his lungs sounded worse. It had only been a couple of hours.

As she turned to go call Dr. Summers, she heard two voices coming down the hall. One was Julia Summers. The other voice was Dr. Sneed. Sara waited and listened.

"This could be a good opportunity to for some lung biopsies. We could probably get wonderful pathology pictures for my next presentation in Canada." she heard Dr. Sneed tell Julia.

"I don't know if the owners will be willing to go that far, Dr. Sneed. This horse has really gone down in the last couple of hours. I don't know if he will be strong enough for the procedure. I think the owners' will want to know about the tests we ran this morning before we do any more procedures. Besides, we can always get the lung biopsies if the horse dies." Julia responded.

"Well, that's true, but I would also really like to get them before. We don't know that the owner won't come pick up the horse's body, and if they do that, we've lost our chance."

Sara didn't hear any response from Julia, but she knew what she thought about Dr. Sneed's plan. A biopsy was going to tell them that Quincy's lungs were diseased. They already knew that. A biopsy was going to tell them that Quincy's had pneumonia and what kind of organisms was causing the pneumonia. They already knew he had pneumonia, and the chances were strong that the transtracheal was would tell them exactly what kind of organism was involved.

It would take days to get the results of a lung biopsy back, and if Quincy kept going down, he didn't have days. There was one reason Sara could think of that Dr. Sneed wanted a lung biopsy and one reason only - for his presentation.

Sara felt her exhaustion and worry over Quincy melt away. She became very calm - too calm. A white, hot light had started in her brain and was working it's way down the rest of her body. That light was anger, and Sara felt it spread in her like a wave that couldn't be stopped.

She clenched her teeth and then she clenched her fist. She was still eerily calm - a kind of calm she only got when she was very angry. The vein in the middle of her forehead actually throbbed. Sara didn't care who Timothy Sneed was. No one was hurting her horse. The world fell away, and Sara saw the source of her anger enter Quincy's stall.

Chapter 47

"Well, hello, there. Hear this boy isn't doing so well." Dr. Sneed said to Sara, as he started placing his stethoscope up to his ears.

"No, sir, he's not." Replied Sara.

The intensity of her answer made Timothy Sneed stop and look at Sara.

This did not look like the same student he vaguely remembered from four days ago. That student had looked down when he spoke. That student had done her best to stay out of his way. This was a different person he saw across the stall now.

She had to be tired, he reasoned. He knew the treatment schedule for this horse, but this student didn't look tired. She looked ready for a marathon. He noticed the clenched jaw and the clenched fist. She was taking even, measured steady breaths, and her nostrils flared every time she inhaled. Her eyes were slits of fire and those eyes were looking directly at him. Her head was held high and back with her chin tilted upwards in what he thought may be defiance. He was a lot taller than this student, but at this moment, he didn't feel it. He could swear she was looking down at him, and besides her reply to him, she had not said another word.

Most students, when he decided to grace them with his presence, either stayed out of his way or tried small talk. He knew he intimidated them, and he meant to. His rotations in the clinic were required by his job. He detested them. They took time away from more important things like research and fund raising.

Timothy Sneed knew he took his dislike for the clinical rotations out on the students, but he didn't care. It brightened this otherwise dreary task. He always felt a nice, little jolt of power when the students cringed under his presence. This student, however, was not cringing.

Dr. Sneed did know Sara. He didn't really remember her name, but he had been briefed by Dr. Summers about her. He knew she was bright and hard working. He knew she had done a fine job on this rotation, and even though his reports from Dr. Summers had been that Sara got along well with other students, interns, and residents, he felt that if he pushed Sara today, he might see another side of this student. In fact, as he glanced her way, again, he was sure of it.

He decided to let it go. She had neither said nor done anything disrespectful, and he had much more important things to do today than look at this horse and antagonize this student. He put the stethoscope to his ears and began to listen to Quincy's lungs.

Julia Summers had taken this all in. She felt like a person watching a very tense silent movie. When they had entered the stall, and she had seen Sara, she knew Sara had heard them talking in the hall. Sara was very composed, but Julia had never seen such effort from Sara to stay composed as she was seeing today. She prayed that Dr. Sneed just examined the horse and got out of there. She did not want a scene with this student and this man. It would not turn out well for Sara, and that would break Julia Summers' heart.

Sara watched the great Dr. Sneed examine Quincy. She wanted him to question her. She wanted him to tell her his plans for Quincy. Even though she knew she would have to be very careful with him, it could mean her veterinary career; she wanted to confront this man, this so-called veterinarian.

Dr. Sneed had forgotten what his career was really about, and he was not going to use her horse for research or to further his career. He was not going to put her horse through painful and potentially harmful tests that in the end would probably tell them nothing. Sara didn't even want him touching Quincy. As far as she was concerned, this man did not have a tenth of the heart or the courage of her horse, and Sara wanted him as far away from Quincy as possible. She waited, patiently, quietly, and angrily as Timothy Sneed finished his exam of Quincy.

"I think the earliest we could get that lung biopsy would be in the morning. What do you think about the scheduling, Dr. Summers?" Dr. Sneed asked.

Sara glared at him. She never turned to acknowledge Dr. Summers at all. She wished her stare were a laser beam that would blow Timothy Sneed to pieces.

"I'm not sure. I'll call surgery and see." Dr. Summers replied.

Julia Summers then turned her eyes to Sara and willed her to look at her. Sara felt the pleading glance of Julia Summers and their eyes met.

"The clients would have to approve the procedure, though. I'm not sure they would." Dr. Summers said. "What do you think, Sara?"

Sara and Julia were reading each others minds and if Timothy Sneed had any insight into women, he would have known, too. Julia was pretty sure Sara could talk Judy Taylor out of the biopsy, and Dr. Sneed would never have to know. The women had a plan that included keeping both Quincy and Sara's career safe, and they had never spoken a word.

"I'll talk to her about it when I call this afternoon." Sara replied.

"Okay, then, we have a plan. I'll talk with you this afternoon, Dr. Summers." Dr. Sneed replied as he left the stall. He took one more glance back at the student. She was still staring at him with what he was sure was total contempt and anger, but she had not spoken a disrespectful word. He didn't have time to worry about it. He needed to get back to his office, and back to his research.

Julia Summers looked at Sara and sighed.

"I don't want to know about your and Mrs. Taylor's conversations. You do what you have to do for your horse and your peace of mind."

Sara nodded with complete respect to Dr. Summers.

"You've still got about fifteen minutes before lunch. Grab yourself something to eat, and I'll meet you back up front for the afternoon patients."

Sara nodded again, and Julia Summers left.

Sara stayed with Quincy for another minute or two. She held his big, sweaty neck and whispered words of encouragement to him. Her anger was subsiding, and she knew without a doubt, that Julia

Summers was behind her. Dr. Sneed would not be doing unnecessary procedures on Quincy. The women would make sure of that.

Sara gave Quincy one last scratch on his head, and when she did, he glanced sideways at her. He was coming out of the sedation, but he still looked bad. As Sara left the stall, she heard him softly nicker. She turned around, and the big old horse stumbled up to her and put his head on her shoulder.

"I love you, too, Quincy. I love you, too."

The horse and the woman stayed that way a couple more minutes. Then Quincy turned and went to the corner of his stall. Sara blew him a sad kiss and went to talk to Dr. Butler before afternoon appointments.

Chapter 48

"Come in, Sara, come in." Dr. Butler welcomed Sara into his office. "You excited about the Ames trip?"

"Well, Dr. Butler, that's what I came to talk to you about. I may not be able to go." Sara looked dejected.

"Really, Sara, why not?" His brows creased in concern. Dr. Harry Butler knew Sara well - well enough to know that she wanted to go on the trip and well enough to know that if she was turning the trip down, something was wrong.

"I'm taking care of a horse on the medicine rotation, and he has taken a turn for the worse. I just don't think it's a good idea for me to leave him." Sara bit her lip and looked down waiting for his reply.

"There are other students on the rotation that can take care of the horse, aren't there, Sara?" Dr. Butler knew there were other students who would be assigned the horse when Sara went to Ames. Something else was keeping her here.

"Yes, sir, there are, but this horse is kind of quirky and won't let just anyone take care of him. He prefers me." Sara replied.

Dr. Butler noticed that the tip of Sara's nose was turning red and her eyes hinted at the real possibilities of tears.

"You okay, Sara?" Dr. Butler genuinely asked.

"Yes, sir." Sara's voice quivered.

Harry Butler had seen this student castrate and dehorn cattle without flinching. He had watched Sara and admired her skill with rectal palpation and ultrasound for pregnancy checking. One day, he and Sara had delivered two calves at the same farm five minutes apart. He had delivered one while Sara delivered the other.

She had been cool and calm under pressure and performed beautifully. When they had left that day, Sara had been covered in afterbirth, blood, and manure. They had stopped at a convenience store on the way back for cokes. Sara had walked in, got her drink, and paid like she was clean and dressed for a date. The patrons of the store had been shocked at her appearance. She hadn't even acted like she had noticed.

That same student was standing before him now with tears in her eyes telling him that she was not going on a trip that he knew she had hoped for all year.

"Why aren't you going then?" He asked quietly.

She looked up and looked him in the eyes and replied, "I can't leave this horse."

He had seen that same look from Sara on the day they were delivering the calves. The calves were big, too big. The calves had started as embryos from a large, muscled beef breed. They had been implanted into Holsteins, a milking breed, to grow and be delivered. Most Holsteins could spit out a beef calf and not even miss a step, but the owner had made a miscalculation with these calves. He had placed them in Holsteins that had never had calves before and both the heifers were having trouble. The calves had grown large. They were expensive calves and it was very important, financially, that the calves be born alive.

He had just been finishing up on his cow and calf when he had glanced over to Sara delivering her calf not ten feet away. She seemed to be struggling.

"You need some help over there, Sara?" He had asked.

She had both arms in the cow up to her shoulder. Her face was nearly touching the cow's rear end and had been turned away from him. At the offer of help, she had turned her face back to him while she manipulated the calf inside the cow.

He had seen the look then - the look of determination as Sara had declined his help and told him she was just fine. He just needed to give her a minute, please.

He had given Sara the time, and she had done her job. He realized as she stood there with that look on her face, he needed to give her this time, too, and let her do this job, the horse, instead of going to Ames. They would be short a student, but that was okay. Even if he insisted, he knew Sara would resist. He had no doubt in his mind that Sara wanted to go to Ames, but whatever was going on with this horse, she was going to see it to the end. He respected her for that - for that and more. Sara would stay.

"I understand, Sara, and it's okay - don't worry about it. If things get better or change, you know you have a place tomorrow. If you're on the van, I'll know you're going. If you're not, I'll know you've had to stay. Sound okay with you?" Dr. Butler asked.

Sara smiled a thankful smile to Dr. Butler. He understood. Sara knew he would, and she was so thankful that most of her professors and clinicians had been like Dr. Butler instead of Dr. Sneed. The contrast was never more than standing in the doorway of this man's office. He could have insisted she go and made life very hard on her if she didn't, but he chose not to. He knew she wouldn't miss the Ames trip for the world, but right now, her world was Quincy, and she was not going to leave him.

"Sounds great, Dr. Butler. Thank you." Sara told Harry Butler.

"You're welcome, Sara. Hang in there."

Sara nodded. "Yes, sir, I will." As Sara left Dr. Butler's office, she heard him say to himself, "No doubt in my mind you will, Sara."

She smiled again, took a deep breath, and made her way down to the clinics for afternoon patients.

Chapter 49

The afternoon went much like the morning. Sara saw several patients and did not have to hospitalize one. The great practitioner was at least looking out for her on this. She could concentrate on Quincy.

He was the same at the two o'clock treatment. By three, in between patients, Sara had checked his chart. His bloodwork, x-ray, and part of the transtracheal wash results were in. None looked hopeful. His lungs were worse and the hateful little bug that was causing the pneumonia, as the bloodwork and x-rays confirmed, was not backing down. It was winning.

What was more concerning was the fact that the transtracheal wash had recovered the hateful bacteria and so far, the bacteria was not showing sensitivity to any of the antibiotics they had tried in the lab. Preliminary results showed it was resistant to most antibiotics, even the ones they were using. Quincy had probably gotten better because he had a mixed infection of different bacteria. The antibiotics they were using had been successful on these bacteria while the resistant bacteria had just been sitting there waiting for the others to die off. When they had, it had flourished. They had to find an antibiotic that would kill it. If they couldn't, it would kill Quincy.

With her test results in hand, Sara went off to find Dr. Summers. Julia was with Doug outside one of the other exam rooms discussing a case. Sara walked up and waited patiently.

"So, I think that should cover it, Doug." Dr. Summers was saying.

"Yes, ma'am, me, too. I think we should probably re-check the goat in one week, though, don't you?" asked Doug.

"Your patient, Doug. Make a decision. Should we re-check or not?"

"I think we need to know what it's bloodwork looks like after a week of treatment."

"Your patient, Doug." Replied Julia.

"Okay, I'm going for the re-check, then." Doug smiled to Dr. Summers.

"Sounds good to me. See you in rounds at four." Replied Julia.

Doug nodded at Sara as he went back into the exam room. He already had sympathy in his eyes, and Sara knew that her group had probably talked among themselves today about Sara and about Quincy. She loved her classmates, and she needed their support. None of them would ask her about Quincy. They knew she didn't want to talk about it, but all of them would be there for her, if she needed them. Sara was thankful.

Sara turned to Dr. Summers, "Did you see the results?"

"Yes, Sara, I did."

"I don't know what to do." Sara said pleadingly to Dr. Summers.

"Sara, I'm not sure there is a lot we can do. We will talk at rounds about different choices and combinations of antibiotics and decide what the best course for Quincy will be. I need to talk to Dr. Sneed about the results, and I need to think. I'll have an answer for you by four, okay?"

"Okay." Sara was relieved. Dr. Summers was taking over. Sara had done all she could do but hopefully Dr. Summers' experience and expertise along with her more advance education would come in handy. As far as Sara was concerned, they should even entertain ideas from Dr. Sneed - as long as they were helpful ideas. He had more experience, expertise, and education than she and Dr. Summers together. Sara just didn't want any unnecessary and or painful tests done on Quincy.

"By the way, Sara, have you talked to Mrs. Taylor?"

"We're done with patients, yes?" asked Sara.

"Yes."

"I'm on my way now. Thanks Dr. Summers."

"Sure, Sara, no problem.

Chapter 50

Sara went outside and got her cell phone out of her pocket. She didn't want to use one of the phones in the clinic. Sara walked to the area where she always grazed Quincy. It was quieter here, and it was peaceful. She would be able to hear Judy better, and she would be able to think. Sara dialed the number, and Judy answered on the second ring.

"Hello."

"Hello, Mrs. Judy - it's Sara. We have some test results." Sara said.

"Okay, Sara, I'm ready. Go ahead. Tell me what we're looking at." Judy waited holding her breath.

"Preliminary findings show a probable resistant bacteria that has overgrown in his lungs making his pneumonia much worse. His bloodwork also looks bad, Mrs. Judy." Sara paused but Judy said nothing.

She continued, "We are hoping that a different combination of antibiotics may help kill this bacteria, and we are going to start them as soon as I get off the phone with you." Sara paused again. Judy still did not speak.

"We're hoping to see improvement by the morning, Mrs. Taylor, and Dr. Sneed also wants you to think about having a lung biopsy done on Quincy." This time it was Sara who did not speak. She waited for Judy to respond.

"A lung biopsy? Why would we do that, and how would that help?" Asked Judy.

"Well, it would probably tell us for sure the bacteria we are dealing with although the wash is pretty accurate, and it would tell us how damaged Quincy's lungs are from his disease and this pneumonia." Sara waited.

"We already know his lungs are badly damaged, don't we, Sara? We've been fighting this for years!" Judy exclaimed.

"Yes, ma'am, we do." Sara plainly stated.

"If we did the biopsy, how long would it take to isolate the bug, and do you think he's strong enough for the procedure? If we think we already know for sure what bacteria it is, wouldn't this just be a waste of time and money?" Judy asked strongly.

Now it was time for Sara to inhale and take a breath. If she answered Judy's questions the way she wanted to, she could get in big trouble if Mrs. Taylor spoke with Dr. Sneed. If she answered Judy's questions the way Dr. Sneed wanted her to, Quincy would go through a painful procedure with limited benefit. Sara exhaled and answered Judy's questions.

"It would probably take several days to grow the bacteria from the lung tissue, and it can take longer to positively identify the bacteria and any antibiotics it may be sensitive to. We think this is a resistant strain that may not be sensitive to any. I do not think Quincy is strong enough to go through the procedure. I think one of the reasons he has this aggressive, weird bacteria is because his immune system and his lungs are weak. I, personally, do not think this procedure will help us, and if he were my horse," Sara paused, "If he were my horse, THERE IS NO WAY I'd put him through it."

She waited for Judy's reply.

"Do what you think is best, Sara. I trust you. I've heard from you every day and most days, more than once. I have not talked to Dr. Sneed since the day I left Quincy. You do what you have to do, and you just keep me informed." Judy commanded.

"I will." Sara replied.

Both women were silent on the phone. Sara could sense Judy wanted to say more or had other questions.

"What is it, Mrs. Taylor?" Sara asked.

"We're going to lose him, aren't we, Sara?" Judy asked.

Both women were silent on the phone. Sara swallowed hard and honestly answered Judy Taylor's question.

"Yes, ma'am. I think we are." The tears came again. They welled up in Sara's eyes as she admitted for the first time in four days that the chances were very much against Quincy ever walking out of the University of Tennessee College of Veterinary Medicine Large Animal Clinic.

"Don't let him suffer, Sara." Judy replied.

"If he's not better in the morning, Mrs. Taylor, we need to have a very serious talk." Sara could not believe those words were coming out of her mouth, but deep down, she knew what she would see when she went to Quincy's stall at rounds. He would be worse. The clinical voice had told her all along but she had chosen not to listen. Her heart would not let her.

Now, her heart saw Quincy very sick again, and it was ready to listen. If Quincy couldn't get better with the new antibiotics, he wasn't going to get better, and Sara wouldn't have him suffer any longer. She wanted to give the other antibiotics a chance, but if Quincy continued to go downhill, he would be much worse by morning, and it would be time.

"I know, Sara. Let's give him tonight, and if he's worse in the morning, we'll talk about it then. I'll be waiting for your call in the morning."

"Yes, ma'am."

"Take care of my boy, Sara."

Sara paused, a tear rolled down her cheek, her voice cracked "I will, Mrs. Taylor, I will."

Sara hung up the phone and checked her watch. She had fifteen minutes before rounds, and she needed to compose herself. She looked out over the grass to Chapman highway. People were carrying their kids' home from school and driving home from work. It was just another day.

A young mother with two small children stopped at the red light by one of the entrances into the college. She and her children were singing and laughing while they sat in the car. Sara wondered, only for a moment, did she take the wrong path? The mother didn't look much older than Sara, and she looked so happy. Her children looked happy, too.

Is that what I should be doing? Should I be looking for a husband and thinking about having kids instead of this? It's just another day for them, coming home from school. I'm on four days straight without hardly any sleep, any food, and in anguish about a horse that's not even mine. I'm exhausted, hungry, stressed, and devastated about a horse. Even if he does get better and go home, there will be more. There will be many more. What am I doing?

Sara turned to go back into the clinic. She walked to Quincy's stall. He didn't even acknowledge she was there. It was all he could do to breath. Sweat had now began to form small puddles around his front legs, and he was breathing exactly the same way he had when he had struggled to walk in the exam room four days ago.

Sara walked up to him and stood. Sadness and despair overwhelmed her. She didn't say a word. She just stood there.

Quincy still did not look up at her but took two wobbly steps and pushed his head to her chest. Sara stroked both sides of his face and began to coo soft words to this sick horse.

All doubts went away. This was exactly where she was supposed to be, and this was exactly who she was supposed to be. If she couldn't make him better, she would make sure he was as comfortable as she could make him. She did not belong, at this time in her life, in a car singing with her children. She belonged here. She knew there would be many more. That's why she was here, but she also knew there would only be one Quincy.

Chapter 51

"Hey, Sara, we're here." Josh spoke softly.

Sara turned to all her classmates standing outside the stall. She had not heard them approach, but they were there. Even Stephanie was there. They were all waiting quietly, patiently for rounds to begin. They had not wanted to disturb Sara and Quincy. Even Dr. Summers was there, and softly she began.

"Okay, as we can all see, Quincy is not doing well. Sara, please go over what we did today for Quincy, his results, and I'll talk about the changes we are making to his treatment regimen." Dr. Summers said.

Sara went over the test, the results, and his prognosis. She talked about the resistant bacteria, and their plan for combination antibiotics, pain relievers, and breathing treatments. Dr. Summers talked about the different antibiotics and the changes in his treatment. Sara would now treat Quincy every four hours with several different combination antibiotics to get his infection under control. He would also have a continuous antibiotic drip as well as the intravenous fluids. As they neared the end of the discussion, Sara had one last question for Dr. Summers.

"When do we talk to the clients about euthanasia?"

"If he's not better at all in the morning, I think that would be a good time."

The whole group was silent.

"Are we still considering the other test?" asked Sara.

"Dr. Sneed is pushing pretty hard, Sara." Dr. Summers replied.

"Judy does not want any further tests done on Quincy." Sara reported.

"Dr. Sneed is gone for the day, but he will probably want to call and talk with her in the morning. He usually comes in around nine or so, but we'll reevaluate in the morning."

"Yes, ma'am." Sara looked into Julia's eyes. Julia was smart, but she was also slick. She knew Sara would call Judy well before nine in the morning. As Sara had thought earlier, Julia was on her and Quincy's side. Julia had everything worked out without Dr. Sneed knowing a thing and without a word being spoken. Sara wondered who the real genius was and smiled at her resident.

Julia smiled back. "Sara, go ahead and get Quincy started on his new treatments and then catch up with us. Stephanie's here to help you."

Sara nodded.

"Okay, guys, let's get going. Daylight's burning." As the students and Dr. Summers made their way to other patients, Stephanie and Sara worked on Quincy.

"He looks bad, Sara." Stephanie noted.

"Yes, he does, Stephanie. I'm not so sure he doesn't look worse than when he came in. Every time I've checked in on him today except once, he looks like he's going downhill. His temperature is still climbing, and his breathing is worse. I hope these antibiotics do the job." Sara tried to keep all doubt from her voice.

"I hope they do to, Sara." Replied Stephanie. They did the rest of their work in silence. It didn't take long. Quincy never moved while they hung the i.v. antibiotics and piggy-backed them into his fluids. He never made a step as they gave two large shots of antibiotics into his rump. He never lifted his head for the breathing treatment. He just stood there and tried to breathe as the sweat continued to roll off of him and his wheezing seemed to get louder in small increments with every breath.

As they finished, and Sara started to leave to catch up with rounds, Stephanie asked, "You'll be checking on him most of the night, I figure?"

"Yes." Sara said resolutely.

"If you need any help, call me. I don't care what time, okay?"

Sara nodded, "Thanks, Stephanie. You don't know how much I appreciate that."

"It's my job, Sara." Stephanie said with a sad smile. "I'll be here if they need me."

"Does it get easier, Stephanie?" Sara asked with complete sincerity.

"I don't think it gets easier, I think we just get more used to it. We love them - that's why we do it, but it takes a toll. I'm not going to lie to you." Stephanie continued, "You hate it for the animal, but you hate it for the people, too. It's almost like veterinarians treat the animals, but a lot of times, they end up treating the people, too. They treat them with their words, and their sympathy, and their caring. It's hard, but it's rewarding, and you do get more used to it after awhile, I promise. Sometimes, the first ones are the hardest ones, Sara."

"They are worth it, though, aren't they." Sara replied as a statement, not a question.

"Yes, they are. They have only their owners and us. They can't tell us what's wrong; you have to figure it out. They may kick and bite, but they don't back talk, and their emotions are always true." Stephanie smiled at Sara.

"Thanks, Stephanie."

"Call me if you need me."

Sara nodded as she left to catch up with her other classmates in rounds, but she kept hearing Stephanie's words in her head through rounds. She was glad Dr. Summers did not call on her. For the first time since clinical rotations began, Sara was not paying attention.

"Their emotions are always true - their emotions are always true - their emotions are always true."

Chapter 52

Rounds were over. Sara returned promptly to Quincy's stall. Leanne was waiting for her there.

"He looks awful, Sara." Leanne stated.

"I know."

"You're not going to Ames, are you? You can't, can you?"

"No, I can't leave him."

Both of the girls looked at the horse in front of him. Sara could swear he even looked worse than he had minutes ago. He was going downhill fast, and her heart was breaking.

"I understand. Tell you what, though. Why don't you tell me what you would pack if you were going, and I'll go ahead and get it packed just in case you get to go?" Leanne asked shyly.

"I'm not going, Leanne." Sara replied sternly.

"Sara, you know as well as I do that Quincy may not make it through the night or past in the morning. Tell me what you want me to pack - just in case - and let me handle it. If things do go wrong, you're going to want out of here, okay? Please." Leanne pleaded.

Sara sighed and looked at Quincy. Leanne was right. Sara needed to make plans, just in case.

"Okay, this is what I'll need..." and Sara gave Leanne a list of things she would need if she went to Ames.

When she finished, Sara gave Leanne a hug. "I really appreciate you, neighbor."

"I know, but don't get too worked up. I'm only doing this because Bubbles will definitely need someone when I'm on small animal intensive care." Leanne smiled.

"Okay, whatever."

Leanne patted Sara on the back. "Hang in there. I'll take care of the home front."

Sara nodded, hugged Leanne again, and waved goodbye to her as her friend turned and headed home.

Sara turned back to Quincy in the stall, went in and set down beside the door.

"I think it's going to be a long night, Buddy."

Quincy never looked up.

Chapter 53

Sara had set there in the stall with Quincy for two hours. She had monitored his ivs, his breathing, his respiration rate, his temperature, and his pulse. All of his vitals were worsening, and he needed pain medication more frequently. He cared nothing about hay, grain, or treats, and he had not moved from the same spot the entire time Sara had been with him.

Around seven, Sara decided to pick up some books from the library and get some quick supper from the vending machines. She was back in his stall by the eight o'clock treatment.

Sara continued with more antibiotics, more pain relievers, and more breathing treatments. Quincy continued to get worse. By ten o'clock, Sara wasn't sure he was going to make it to the morning. His temperature had climbed to 104 degrees, even with medications. His breathing was quick and shallow and his mucus membranes began to take on a distinct blue hue.

Oddly enough, she did not feel a tremendous amount of emotion. She was machine like in her treatments. She did not stand by him for him to step up to nuzzle her - he didn't have the strength, and she knew it. He was doing everything he could to breathe and keep his heart beating. She would stroke and pet him when she treated him, but then she would leave him alone and go back to the book she had picked up at the library.

His eyes were different, and Sara had seen this earlier in the night. There was no fire left in them now, there was no pleading. He, like Sara, was empty now, and both the woman and the horse went about their business. Sara's business was to make Quincy as comfortable as she could with the very small glimmer of hope that any minute, the antibiotics were going to start making him feel better. Quincy's business was to continue to breathe.

Some of her classmates trickled by through the night to give Sara words of encouragement. She smiled and said thank you, but their words fell on deaf ears. Quincy was all but gone, and Sara had accepted that fact. She didn't know when, but somehow, she had. She was empty. She felt nothing. She was numb.

After the four a.m. treatment, Sara returned to her sitting place in Quincy's stall, and again, began to read. She heard Quincy move and looked up. He was making his way toward her. It was all he could do to walk.

"Whoa, son, steady. You don't have to come over here. You stay right where you are." Sara said gently. She did not get up but sit right where she was and watched this horse she loved come to her.

Quincy stopped when he got to Sara. His head was down and over the opened book. Sweat began to hit the pages of the book like a slow, summer rain. Sara didn't care. She would pay for the stupid book. It wasn't the safest thing in the world for a sick, wobbly horse that might fall at any minute to be standing over you, but Sara didn't care. If that's where Quincy wanted to be, that's where Quincy would be. She reached up and stroked his soft muzzle.

"I love you, Buddy."

Chapter 54

Dr. Julia Summers arrived at the clinics at six a.m. She knew what she would find, but she was hoping against hope, she was wrong. She wasn't.

As she approached the stall, she saw the big horse with his head down by the stall door. Sara was nowhere in sight. She was surprised - until she got closer.

Inside the stall, Sara was asleep. Quincy stood over her. The book in Sara's lap was soaking wet.

Julia knew she should reprimand Sara heavily for sleeping in Quincy's stall. It wasn't the sleeping. Everyone got little catnaps between treatments. Even in the intensive care units, one could sleep for ten to fifteen minutes between checking their patients. It was sleeping in the horse's stall. One could get hurt badly in a split second with a sick horse.

Julia also knew she would not reprimand Sara. She just couldn't. She rarely saw this type of devotion. She was going to keep her mouth shut.

Julia cleared her throat, and Sara woke up.

"Oh, sorry, Dr. Summers. I didn't hear you." Sara moved Quincy's head and stood up. She couldn't believe she had fallen asleep like that. She was worried what Dr. Summers would say, but Julia didn't say a word except to ask about Quincy.

"He's worse." Sara flatly answered.

"I see that, Sara. I'm so sorry." Julia replied, and she truly was. When someone had been doing this job as long as Julia, not much got to you, but this student and this horse had found their way into her gritty heart, and she was sorry for all involved - Quincy, Sara, and Judy Taylor.

"I think maybe you need to call Mrs. Taylor, Sara, and let her know how he's doing. Is his temp down any?" Julia asked.

"No ma'am. It's stayed between 104 and 106 all night. He's not any better. He can hardly walk, and he's getting pain meds every hour. The antibiotics are not working." Sara reported.

"Go call her, Sara." Julia said with a sigh.

Yes, ma'am." Sara replied as she exited the stall and headed for the phones.

Judy answered on the first ring.

"He's not better, Mrs. Taylor. He's worse." Sara reported with no emotion.

"Is he suffering, Sara?" Judy asked.

"Yes, ma'am. I gave him pain meds every hour on the hour through the night to help him through. I was hoping the antibiotics would kick in and get him going again, but it's been over twelve hours with no change. " Sara replied.

"Sara, if he were your horse, what would you do?" Judy asked slowly, intently.

"Mrs. Judy, we have given him everything we have. He has given us everything he has. I told you I wouldn't let him suffer, but he has been suffering since last night, and I'm sorry. I just thought maybe we could give him one more chance, and it would be worth it. I thought maybe the medicine would work. I was wrong. He is tired, Mrs. Judy. He's ready. If he were mine, I'd put him down. He's been through enough." Sara felt a tickle in her throat as she spoke to Mrs. Taylor. Her stomach began to tighten and that huge, empty, nothing feeling began to go away.

There was a long silence on the phone. Judy spoke in broken words and sobs as she asked, "Is it fair to him to wait until I get there, Sara? Can we do that?"

"Mrs. Judy," Sara paused. The nothing feeling was slowly being eaten away with sadness and grief. "We can keep him alive until you get here, but that's at least six to seven more hours, and honestly, it wouldn't be fair to him. We've done all we can do. He's your horse. We'll do what you want, though."

There was another long pause between the two women. Sara could hear Judy crying in the background. She finally composed herself enough to speak, "Go ahead, Sara. Let my boy rest. Let him sleep."

With those words, the emptiness completely vanished. The tickle in Sara's throat had become like a vice choking the breath from her, and the tears started to form for what seemed to Sara like the thousandth time over the last twenty-four hours.

"I love Quincy, Mrs. Taylor, and we will make sure your boy goes to sleep comfortably. We will take good care of him. We will be done within the hour." Sara could hardly choke out the words. "I just want you to know it has been an honor and a pleasure to work for you and with Quincy. I'll never forget him."

"I know, Sara, and neither will I. Thank you so much for all you've done. You'll never know how much we appreciate it."

"You're welcome, Mrs. Taylor."

"We'll be to get him this afternoon, Sara. We are burying him on the farm."

"Yes, ma'am. I'll let them know."

"Good-bye, Sara."

"Good-bye, Mrs. Judy."

Sara hung up the phone and took a minute to compose herself. She thought she was past this. Last night had seemed like a dream. She had accepted this and made peace with herself and with Quincy. Where was all this emotion coming from? Sara didn't know, but emotion was welling up in her like an ocean, and she was fighting with all her might to keep the waves down. She had a job to do. She needed to get control.

Sara breathed several deep breaths. She thought of home. She thought of anything but Quincy, and finally, slowly but surely, she calmed down. She went to the bathroom, blew her nose and washed her face. She felt better now. She was ready to face this terrible day.

Chapter 55

As Sara walked out of the bathrooms and down the hall, she noticed Doug coming out of the break room. He usually wasn't here this early. As she walked further down the hall, she saw Hillary slipping in the back door. Josh followed, then Jessica. They were all at least an hour early, and they were all headed for Quincy's stall.

Sara and her classmates arrived at Quincy's stall together. Dr. Summer's was waiting. No one said a word. They all knew the padded room they were taking Quincy to. It had big doors and easy access to the outside. They all looked at each other in unison, and Sara grabbed Quincy's halter and lead rope. Dr. Summers opened the stall door for Sara.

Quincy was now sweating so profusely that his bedding was a wet slush beneath him. You could hear him breathe down the hall. His eyes were dull and lifeless, and he looked like he had lost a hundred pounds in twenty-four hours.

Sara placed the halter on Quincy, and disconnected his iv line. She clucked for him to follow. He did not move. She clucked again and pulled on the lead rope harder. He took a few stumbling steps and nearly fell. He was not strong enough to walk out of the stall. He wanted to mind Sara, but he was so weak, he could not balance. The bacteria had more than taken its toll through the night.

"Doug, you and Josh get behind him and help him balance." Dr. Summers motioned to the boys.

Sara again clucked to Quincy as the boys pushed him from the back. Hillary and Jessica moved to his sides. He cleared the stall but then almost fell. It was torture.

Sara saw quickly that Doug and Josh did not know how to balance a horse using its tail. They only knew how to push. They were both strong and when they pushed, Quincy could not keep up with their strength on his front end. Sara knew how to balance a horse using its tail. She hadn't learned that from a book. She had learned it at the animal clinic at home.

"Dr. Summers, why don't you let me get in back with the guys, and Hillary can lead him?" Sara pleaded.

The women nodded, and Sara moved to Quincy's tail. She raised it, and on the next push/pull, she helped him balance. This time, he kept his balance much better. He was stumbling, but he was not falling. They helped Quincy take a step or two, and then they let him rest. They continued down the hall this way - two steps, balance, and rest.

The room was not more than twenty feet away, but to Sara, it seemed a mile away, and as the group did everything they could to help this horse move and to keep him from falling, Sara realized three things: Her classmates were there to help, Dr. Summers was making sure Dr. Sneed would not talk Judy Taylor into the test he wanted to run, and Quincy was taking his last walk.

Tears did not just well up in Sara's eyes. She had been fighting them now on and off for days. She could fight them no longer. Sara Caldwell began to cry, and tears began to stream down her cheeks like a river that has finally been set free. Sara could not remember the last time she had cried, but oh my goodness, how she was crying today.

With tears streaming down her face and neck, Sara urged Quincy on. Her classmates also began urging the big horse on, and he began walking better, faster to the room. When they finally arrived, Dr. Summers signaled her classmates and at once, they all left the room.

"Sara, you want to spend some time with him alone?" Julia Summers asked her student.

Sara was crying so hard, she couldn't speak. She nodded to Julia.

"I'll be right outside. You just let me know when you are ready."

Sara nodded again, and Julia left.

And there they stood, one last time - the horse and the woman. Sara put her arms around Quincy's neck and sobbed. He could barely stand. He was completely wet with sweat, and he could hardly take in any air at all.

Sara stepped back. She could not stand it anymore.

Quincy stepped forward, and Sara stopped.

The once great horse took his head and placed it down on Sara's knee. With all the strength he had left in his body, he slowly rubbed that big head all the way up Sara's body, nearly knocking her down, and left it to rest on her shoulder, just as Judy said he used to do when he was happy.

Sara sobbed. She could feel his ragged breaths in her ear, and then Quincy took a deep breath, let out a long sigh, and stepped back from Sara. He had said his thank you's and his goodbyes. He loved this woman, but he was tired. He knew why they had brought him to this room, and he was thankful. He was ready to sleep, and Sara could see it in his eyes.

Sara nodded to Quincy and on legs she did not feel, went to get Dr. Summers. Julia was waiting outside the door.

"We're ready, Dr. Summers." Sara said.

"Doug and I are going to take care of Quincy, Sara. Dr. Butler is waiting with the group in the van for you to go to Ames. Leanne brought your bag early this morning, and they already have it packed. They are ready for you."

Sara began shaking her head no. "I can't leave him now - no way. I'm staying until the end."

Julia Summers put her hand on Sara's arm, looked into her eyes, and asked, "Do you trust me, Sara?"

Sara did not answer but just looked at Julia with a blank stare.

"Sara, do you trust me?" She asked again.

"Yes, ma'am, I do." Sara answered.

"Then let me handle this for you. You will do this many times in your career, but let me handle Quincy. He won't feel a thing - I promise. I will take good care of him, and you know this." Julia nodded for Sara to agree.

"I will feel guilty if I leave." Sara pleaded with Julia.

"Do you want to see this big man laid down, Sara. Do you really? You don't have to prove anything to Quincy or me. Let me handle this for you. It's the least I can do."

And suddenly, Dr. Summers made sense to Sara. Sara did not want to see Quincy take his last breath. She did not want to see him sedated and laid gently down. She did not want to listen to his heart as it took its last beat. She did not want to see his muscles tremor as he died. She would witness this again and again throughout her career, many being at her hand. There was no reason she had to witness this one. Quincy had said his goodbyes. Dr. Summers was right - he would understand.

Sara nodded back to Dr. Summers. "Okay."

Julia Summers gave Sara Caldwell a hug and said in her ear, "Now get out of here and go get on that van."

Chapter 56

Sara walked onto the van that was going to Ames. Hillary and Seth were there. Dr. Butler was driving. No one said a word. The tears had lightened, but Sara could still feel them trickling down her cheeks. Dr. Butler handed her a tissue, and she took her seat in the van.

It was raining on this spring morning in Knoxville, Tennessee. Sara had barely noticed when she got into the van. Hillary silently handed her a pillow, and as she leaned against the window watching the rain blend with her tears, they pulled out of the University of Tennessee College of Veterinary Medicine onto Chapman Highway.

Traffic was beginning to get busy at this hour of the morning, but Sara didn't notice. It would be a long drive to West Tennessee. West Tennessee - where she was born and raised until she moved to Knoxville. West Tennessee - where Quincy came from. West Tennessee - where she grew up riding horses in the fields and the woods behind her rural home.

As they merged onto I-40 West, Sara's thought of riding horses as a girl. The hum of the rain and the cadence of the van soothed her. All was quiet. Sara's eyes begin to close, and Sara slept. As Sara slept, she began to dream.

She was beside the familiar riverbank. The storm and the fog had completely cleared. The river was quietly bubbling beneath her. She looked on the far bank, and there were no horses. She knew she was dreaming. She stood on the solid, dry bank and let the sounds and sights of the river soothe her. The sun was warm on her face.

For several minutes, she was completely alone, but then, in the distance, she heard several horses whinny. She could hear them galloping toward her. As they crested the hill, she could easily pick out the leader she had seen in her dreams so many times before. He did not seem angry today. As always, he was at the front of the band.

Instead of focusing on the leader, however, Sara's eye was drawn to another horse in the band. He was beautiful, and she had not noticed him in her other dreams. He was huge, standing at least 17 hands. His muscular body was burnished red as was his graceful, long neck and well placed head. His jet black mane and tail stood in contrast to the white markings on all four legs and his big blaze reached from his eyes down to his nose. Sara imagined he caused people to stop and stare with his beauty. She began to smile.

The horses slowed as they got closer to the river, and Sara watched this new addition to the herd. As they walked to the riverbank to take a drink, the leader paid Sara no attention whatsoever. He had no reason to be angry. His herd was complete.

The new horse, the beautiful horse, that Sara barely recognized, bent his gorgeous head down to the river and took a long, slow drink. Sara watched him carefully. He had just run at least a half a mile. His breathing was regular and deep. He had not even broken a sweat. The large, firm muscles in his body rippled as he moved. He slowly brought his head up from his drink and looked at Sara - the river between them.

A woman and a horse stood for a moment. Sara smiled. The horse winked. The leader of the band watched, and the other horses drank. When they had finished, the leader turned back toward the pasture and signaled the band to go. They all turned and galloped off through the pasture, over the hill and out of Sara's sight. Not one horse looked back as Sara watched them with a smile on her face.

The dream faded, and Sara slept a deep, peaceful sleep.

www.ingramcontent.com/pod-product-compliance
Lightning Source LLC
Chambersburg PA
CBHW051804170526
45167CB00005B/1877